North American Health Care Policy in the 1990s

North American Health Care Policy in the 1990s

Edited by

ARTHUR KING
THOMAS HYCLAK
ROBERT THORNTON

Lehigh University, Bethlehem, Pennsylvania, USA

and

SAMUEL McMAHON

Battlecreek Health System, Battlecreek, Michigan, USA

JOHN WILEY & SONS
Chichester · New York · Brisbane · Toronto · Singapore

Other Wiley Editorial Offices

John Wiley & Sons, Inc., 605 Third Avenue,
New York, NY 10158-0012, USA

Jacaranda Wiley Ltd, G.P.O. Box 859, Brisbane,
Queensland 4001, Australia

John Wiley & Sons (Canada) Ltd, 22 Worcester Road,
Rexdale. Ontario M9W 1L1, Canada

John Wiley & Sons (SEA) Pte Ltd, 37 Jalan Pemimpin #05-04,
Block B, Union Industrial Building, Singapore 2057

Library of Congress Cataloging-in-Publication Data

North American health care policy in the 1990s/edited by Arthur King
... [et al.].
p. cm.
Includes bibliographical references and index.
ISBN 0 471 94003 8
1. Medical policy—United States. 2. Medical policy—Canada.
3. Medical policy—Economic aspects—United States. 4. Medical
policy—Economic aspects—Canada. I. King, Arthur E.
RA395.A3N67 1993
362.1'0971—dc20 93-15776
CIP

British Library Cataloguing in Publication Data

A catalogue record for this book is available from the British Library

ISBN 0 471 94003 8

Typeset in 11/13 Palacio by Mathematical Composition Setters Ltd, Salisbury.
Printed and bound in Great Britain by Biddles Ltd, Guildford Surrey.

Dedication

We wish to dedicate the publication of this symposium to the memory of our colleague Richard Herman MD, former Chief of the Department of Radiology at St Luke's Hospital, who died just after the lectures were completed. The conception of the lecture series and symposium began several years ago with a heated discussion between Dick Herman and Art King, who were considering the frustrations of the medical profession with cost-based government regulations which had been recently imposed. Dick was the motivating force at St Luke's who brought the idea to the attention of the administration and then served as their liaison and chief planner for the events. Dick was concerned that providers would lose sight of their basic role as healers in a welter of regulations and concerns for financing care. As a realist, nonetheless, he was keenly aware throughout his career of the need to practise medicine in a world of scarce resources. His concern was for the human imperfections in balancing the two objectives of access to quality care in a cost-conscious setting. We miss his guidance, analyses and kindness.

Contents

	Contributors	ix
	Foreword	xiii
	Introduction	xv
Chapter 1	The morality of efficiency in health care: some uncomfortable implications *Anthony J. Culyer*	1
Chapter 2	The Canadian health care system: a model for America to emulate? *C. David Naylor*	25
Chapter 3	Fairness and feasibility in national health care systems *Mark V. Pauly*	67
Chapter 4	Lessons in long-term care: the benefits of a northern exposure *Robert L. Kane*	91
Chapter 5	Quality assurance in Canada: what are the health professions doing? *Carol Kushner*	111
Chapter 6	Management of human resources in health care: the Canadian experience *Orvill B. Adams*	141

Chapter 7 The cost savings–quality trade-off: empirical evidence of a cost–quality trade-off in the provision of community-based long-term care
Paul N. Rappoport and Arthur E. King 169

Chapter 8 Forces for reforming the US health care system: a review of the cost and access issues
Susan M. Browning 197

Chapter 9 Proposals to reform the US health care system: a critical review
John C. Gaffney, Susan M. Browning and Edward B. Hirshfeld 223

Index 275

Contributors

Orvill B. Adams is a principal in the firm of Curry, Adams and Associates, Inc. (Ottawa, Ontario). He works with public and private sector executives, policy-makers and providers in health education and social services to develop short and long-term plans through research and analysis.

J. Richard Aronson PhD is a professor of economics and the Director, Martindale Center for the Study of Private Enterprise, at Lehigh University (Bethlehem, PA). He conducts research in the areas of tax analysis and pension-funding.

Susan M. Browning MPH is the Director, Health System Reform, American Medical Association (Chicago, IL), who is responsible for policy, strategy implementation, advocacy efforts and outreach activities on health system reform. Her research includes federal/state implementation of reform concepts such as managed competition.

Anthony J. Culyer is a professor of economics, Head of the Department of Economics and Related Studies and Pro-Vice-Chancellor of the University of York (England). He is co-editor of the *Journal of Health Economics* and is a member of the Central Research and Development Committee of the National Health Services.

John C. Gaffney PhD is the Director of the Division of Strategic Policy Planning, American Medical Association (Chicago, IL), and is responsible for maintaining the AMA policy base and designing its socio-economic policy planning process. His primary research focuses on identifying changes in the US health sector and their future impact on medical practice.

Edward B. Hirshfeld JD is the Vice-President of the Health

Law Division, American Medical Association (Chicago, IL) who is responsible for providing counsel to the AMA on health law and information on health law to physicians and the public. He is concerned with the interactions in reform among proposals for cost control, liability laws and physician ethics.

Thomas J. Hyclak PhD is a professor of economics and is an Associate Director of the Martindale Center for the Study of Private Enterprise, at Lehigh University (Bethlehem, PA). His research has investigated US and UK regional employment patterns and their connection to housing markets.

Robert L. Kane MD holds the endowed Minnesota Chair in Long-term Care and Aging at the University of Minnesota School of Public Health (Minneapolis, MN). His special interest is long-term care policy. With his wife, Rosalie, he has studied long-term care for older persons in several countries, including Canada.

Arthur E. King PhD is a professor of economics and Director of the Canadian Studies Program at Lehigh University (Bethlehem, PA). He is an econometrician interested in the application of statistical inference in health care services and comparative economics.

Carol Kushner is Vice-President of Health Concepts (Toronto, Ontario). As a writer and researcher on public policy she has had extensive experience as a consultant to government and outside groups on social policy. She is the co-author of *Second Opinion: What is Wrong with Canada's Health Care System and How to Fix It.*

Samuel M. McMahon MD is Vice-President for Medical Affairs at the Battlecreek Health System (Battlecreek, MI). His line responsibilities include medical staff and chiefs of service, medical education, medical administration, and quality assessment and utilisation management. His medical specialties are internal medicine and pulmonary medicine.

C. David Naylor, MD, DPhil, FRCPC is the Director of the Clinical Epidemiological Unit, Sunnybrook Health Science Centre, and the CEO of the Institute for Clinical Evaluative Sciences (North York, Ontario). A career scientist of the Ontario Ministry of Health, his major research focus has been in the realm of cardiovascular diseases, particularly at the interface of clinical epidemiology and public policy.

Mark V. Pauly PhD is the Bendheim Professor, Chairman and Professor of the Health Care Systems Department, Professor of Insurance and Public Policy and Management at the Wharton School, and Professor of Economics in the School of Arts and Sciences at the University of Pennsylvania (Philadelphia, PA). He is also Director of Research at the Leonard Davis Institute of Health Economics.

Paul N. Rappoport PhD is an associate professor of economics at Temple University (Philadelphia, PA). His research includes economic assessment of child welfare, mental retardation and other human service applications. As a practising econometrician for over 20 years, he has worked for governmental agencies, industry and private foundations.

Robert J. Thornton PhD is a professor of economics, Chairman of the Department of Economics and an Associate Director of the Martindale Center for the Study of Private Enterprise, Lehigh University (Bethlehem, PA). His research interests include collective bargaining in the public sector and forensic economics.

Foreword

Reform of the US health care system is high on the agenda of the Administration of President Clinton. In the lead-up to the presidential election in 1992 as many as three dozen different reform proposals were advocated by groups in the US Congress, in addition to those of the then President Bush and many interest groups and academic commentators. Clearly, analysis and synthesis are necessary to focus debate on the issues raised by this vigorous reform effort.

As editors of the the newly launched journal *Health Economics* we decided to contribute to this debate in a variety of ways. We were delighted when Professor King offered us this collection of papers which contribute much to a better informed policy-making process. A particularly interesting feature of the series is the comparison of the US and Canadian systems of health care organisation. Many authors have examined the Canadian system as a way of controlling the growth of health care expenditure in the USA, but there remains an apparent reluctance on the part of opinion leaders and the general US population both to accept cash limits and to confront explicitly the inherent rationing criteria in all resource allocation processes.

The reform of health care systems is a subject of worldwide interest, and this collection of papers has relevance beyond its North American context. The fundamental differences between centrally funded, state-managed systems and even more bureaucratic systems with mixed and open-ended funding sources permeate all debates about health care reforms worldwide. The issues raised in this book seek to identify the ways in which the twin goals of cost containment and efficiency can be achieved in health care. Like the reform of the US health care system these goals all too often seem as elusive as the Holy Grail!

Alan Maynard and John Hutton
University of York, Battelle and MEDTAP Research Centre, London

Introduction

Arthur King, Thomas Hyclak
and J. Richard Aronson
Department of Economics, Lehigh University, Bethlehem, Pennsylvania, USA

As we enter the last decade of the twentieth century, the health care system of the USA continues to be plagued by two serious problems which show few signs of abating: rapidly escalating costs and limited access to care. The national dialogue about health care policy, including the issues of cost and access, has recently expanded to encompass the ideas of many groups, including employers, the private insurance industry, government-funded programmes, physicians and the academic community.

Quite naturally this dialogue has examined health care systems in other countries. In particular, because of the current heightened awareness by the US public of perceived Canadian successes, it is relevant to make careful comparisons with Canada. Despite a very different system of health care finance, Canada grapples with problems of cost and access similar to those in the USA. Observers in the USA who hold Canada's universal Medicare system in high regard and recommend that the USA adopt similar policies have begun to see that many Canadians have concerns that mirror their own. Concerns on both sides of the border include continued expansion of health care costs and decreased levels of accessibility to high-quality care, either due to waiting lists or lack of insurance coverage. The expanded health policy dialogue has resulted in more productive discussion than ever before, but as of yet no consensus has emerged about the appropriate system to finance care, to expand access to care, to assure quality in care and to control the costs of care.

Currently in the USA, many of these issues are 'hot topics' on the political scene. In November 1991, a special election in Pennsylvania to fill an unexpired Senatorial seat appears to have turned on the perception of Senator Wofford that the voters wanted promises of concrete proposals for entitlement to health insurance. Former President Bush, as part of his re-election campaign, unveiled a health insurance proposal based on tax vouchers and additional tax deductions for private, free market coverage of the un/under-insured. In February 1993, First Lady Hillary Clinton was named head of a task-force to propose reforms in the financing of US health care, within the 100 days promised by President Clinton.

Policy-makers have focused on the interdependence of the health care financing issue with other financial concerns of the electorate. Pennsylvania Governor Casey has promised to increase health care coverage for state residents with no increase in taxes. Many retirees fear financial ruin from the costs of long-term illness, and thus refuse to approve school bond issues and other needed publicly financed projects. Assuaging or solving these well-founded fears would give major voting blocs a different set of premises upon which to base their ballots.

With the co-sponsorship of St Luke's Hospital (Bethlehem, PA) and funding from the Canadian Embassy's Canadian Studies Grants Programme, the Martindale Center for the Study of Private Enterprise organised a series of lectures at Lehigh University to address these issues. The chapters in this volume were drawn from that lecture series with additional invited contributions, and were originally published as a series of articles in the journal *Health Economics*.

The chapters fall into three categories: conceptual issues in the design of national health policy; comparative studies of some of the details of Canadian and American health care; and an overview and critique of the current US situation. The conceptual and empirical issues are blended in moving from discussion of broad principles, through specific aspects of health, to assessments of proposals to reform the US health care system.

The first set begins with a chapter by Tony Culyer, which draws on UK and Canadian experience to highlight the ethical issues raised by using economic criteria in the allocation of resources in national health care programmes. Canadian physician David Naylor continues the discussion with a direct comparison of Canadian and US health care finance and the likely future effects on the nature and level of care provision in the two countries.

The second group begins with Mark Pauly's chapter, which addresses equity issues from a US perspective and outlines the conditions for an equitable and efficient national health insurance programme. This is followed by chapters from Robert Kane, Carol Kushner and Orvill Adams on the Canadian experience with long-term care, quality assurance and medical manpower. Paul Rappoport and Arthur King combine all three of these topics with an empirical study of the trade-off between cost savings and quality in a community-based long-term care setting in the USA.

The final two chapters review the situation in the USA as it now stands and suggest some guidelines for policy-makers who will shape the future of the US health care delivery system. Susan Browning reviews the forces for reforming US health care. John Gaffney, Susan Browning and Edward Hirshfeld provide a comprehensive framework for evaluating proposals for national health care delivery and finance. They describe the criteria and apply them to several proposed reforms for the US system. However, their analytical methods can be applied to determine the feasibility of new proposals for a national system of health care finance.

CHAPTER 1

The morality of efficiency in health care: some uncomfortable implications

Anthony J. Culyer
University of York, UK, and University of Toronto, Ontario, Canada

INTRODUCTION

Whether you find my implications comfortable or not will probably depend in large part on whether you start from where I start, or from somewhere else in the geography of health service ideology. Whichever may be the case, it is plainly important for me to lay out my own points of departure. But I would rather not argue about whether they are the right points than about whether what I infer from them are the right implications. I am not going to draw many specific US–Canadian comparisons, but rather leave these for you to draw for yourselves in the light of the more general considerations that I think one needs to address if one is to form a coherent view about the future of health care delivery and finance in the USA, Canada and the UK, or what one may learn from another.

North American Health Care Policy in the 1990s
Edited by A. King, T. Hyclak, S. McMahon and R. Thornton

Donabedian distinguished two broad but rival ethical bases on which systems of health care finance and provision can be constructed and justified.[1] The first considers access to health care to be essentially similar, in ethical respects, to access to the other good things of life (like food, shelter and the pursuit of leisure activities) which are part of society's reward system. Through legitimate work or legitimate inheritance you acquire legitimate income and legitimate wealth which entitle you to purchase a legitimate share of the available marketed good things in society. The second regards access to health care as a right of citizenship like access to the ballot box or courts of justice, which should not depend in any way on individual income and wealth, though it will necessarily have to depend on the income and wealth of society in general (since resources are limited and health is not the only good thing, so health care is only ever going to receive a finite share of the total) and entitlement will also clearly depend on the conditions of 'membership'. On this latter view, which has also been urged by James Tobin, health care is a 'primary good', though not all goods may be deemed such, so that there is still scope, and possibly substantial scope, for the 'rewards' element to play some role in the ethical vision of those holding the second broad viewpoint.[2] The two views are also commonly associated with a complex of other attitudes towards health care, (issues like the extent to which individuals ought legitimately to bear the consequences of their own ineptitude, defective foresight or lack of material achievement), which I have addressed elsewhere.[3]

My general starting point is the second of these two broad viewpoints, which is also a widely held starting point in European countries, including the UK, and which is also an inherent part of Canadian culture. This has some immediate implications for equity in health care. For example, this viewpoint usually entails that horizontal equity, which is the first of Aristotle's duality, requires that individuals having the same need ought to be treated equally, and that his second, vertical equity, grants individuals with greater needs a greater claim on resources. I do not propose, however, to say much about equity, though I shall have to say quite a bit about 'need'.

With that as background, I want to focus on two main questions and the subsidiary issues (or at least some of them) which they raise. The first of these questions concerns what it means to be efficient, what the ethical justification for efficiency is and, as subsidiary issues, what is implied about 'needs' and whether it is ethical to take account of costs in determining health care resource allocations. The second question relates to the individual relationship between doctor and patient, and what the foregoing implies for that. There are a great many further implications for the design of both the finance and delivery of health care, but I am going to leave these for you to figure out largely for yourselves.

EFFICIENCY

One cannot begin to discuss efficiency (or equity) without talking about objectives. I am going to assume, without much discussion, that the objective of health services is to promote health and, moreover, to do so in such a fashion as to maximise the impact on the nation's health of whatever resources are available to this end. There are some equity side-constraints to this which I shall not address here. Given this objective, and granted that it is an ethical objective, an immediate implication follows: it is ethical to be efficient (and unethical to be inefficient). The term 'efficient' evidently needs unpacking, since much confusion about what it is abounds. There are four mutually consistent definitions,[4] which cumulatively embrace those that go before, whose content can be usefully explored at the same time as their ethical status.

The Morality of Efficiency

The first definition of efficiency is as follows: *Providing only services that are effective in the sense that there is believable evidence that patients will enjoy better health with the interventions than without them*. This is sometimes referred to (especially by clinical epidemiologists) as efficacy or effectiveness. Given an objective, such as returning the patient to normal functioning as speedily as possible, one should therefore seek those combinations of diagnostic procedures, physicians' time, medicines, surgical procedures, inpatient and outpatient care, health service and social service and family caring, and the patient's own time, that are most effective. To use more of any of these resources than is necessary for an effective impact is wasteful and inconsistent with the objective of maximising the impact of resources on health in the community. For, if more than is necessary is used, the excess could have been used at no cost to the patients in question in order to further the health of some other patients. Thus, overall community health (whose maximisation is our postulated ethical imperative) is lower than it need be.

Epidemiologists are constantly reminding us that much medical care has never been subject to systematic scientific testing, that much practice is based on that species of gossip known as the case study, that there is often a strong 'medical signature' in explanations of costly variations in clinical practice, and that the statistical design of much clinical research has in the past left much to be desired.[5–11] Moreover, health care as such is only one of the various determinants of health and it may be marginal at that—at least in global terms. For example, take scarlet fever in England and Wales examined by McKeown.[12] In the 1860s the mortality for children from scarlet fever was higher than that from whooping cough, measles or diphtheria but, as Figure 1.1 shows, the rate was declining before the streptococcus had been identified and, by the time that effective chemotherapy in the form of the early sulphonamides became available, the vast bulk of the death toll had been eliminated. Apart from any spontaneous decline in the virulence of disease, the main factors promoting better health seem to have been better nutrition (possibly) and better hygiene (almost certainly). The activities of the humble apothecary or the prestigious fellows of the Royal College of Physicians were alike

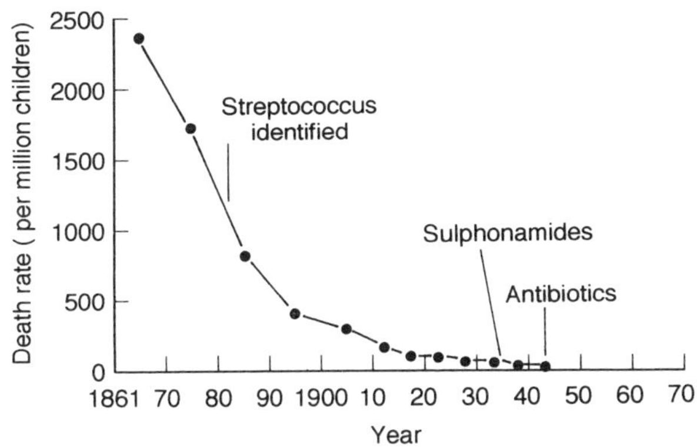

Figure 1.1 Scarlet fever: death rates of children under 15

relatively insignificant, and this seems to have been true of infectious disease generally. I draw these things to your attention not in order to belittle the achievements of scientific medicine—which would be silly—but to draw out two lessons: one factual and one ethical. The factual one is that you cannot take either the absolute or the relative effectiveness of medical practice for granted—it is always reasonable to ask questions about, and to request the evidence for, assertions of effectiveness. The moral one is that to offer ineffective care is unethical, if you allow that maximising the impact of health care on health is a properly moral objective. The reason is simple: resources used on ineffective care, or even only relatively ineffective care, are denied to other purposes that are effective (or more effective)—and that must reduce the overall impact of health care on health.

While this first definition can be used to identify some activities as inefficient, it is not terribly discriminating. There is usually more than one combination of resources represented in more than one method of case management that satisfies the definition. There are substitutions between drugs, between medicine and surgery, between institutional and community care, and so on, which can be made. This gives rise to the great variety of practice that can be observed within areas, between them, and across national boundaries.[13] Although some of these variations may represent ineffective practice, many of them may be equally efficient in the sense of effective. We therefore need a tighter definition, the second meaning of efficiency meets this requirement: *providing whatever services are provided at least resource cost*. This is often called 'cost-effectiveness' and requires the selection from among the effective modes of case management of that which is judged to be least costly. To incur a higher cost than is necessary is again wasteful and inconsistent with the objective of maximising the impact of resources on health in the community. If a higher cost than is necessary is incurred, the excess could have been used at no cost to the patients in question to further the health of some other patients. Thus, overall community health is lower than it need be.

This definition is also insufficiently discriminating. Although it affords a clear criterion for evaluating the efficiency of whatever it is that one is doing so that, for a given expected outcome and other patient-oriented attributes of the procedure, the cost is minimised, it does not tell us whether the procedure is actually worth what it costs and, in particular, whether there are not other programmes of care whose health pay-offs may be higher at the margin (given the resources currently committed to them). The third concept of efficiency deals with this problem: *concentrating resources on those effective services, provided at least cost, which offer the biggest pay-off in terms of health*. Commonly used measures of health pay-offs are reductions in mortality, or survival rates after *x* years, or life-years gained. Since much of modern medicine is not addressed to life-saving but to quality-of-life improving, it seems necessary to recognise the limitations of these views of the productivity of health care and find something more comprehensive and subtle. One instrument that has recently acquired some popularity—and not a little notoriety—is a Canadian invention: the quality-adjusted life-year or QALY.[14] This tool makes explicit assumptions about the relative values of alternative states of health or ill-health which, when applied to expected survival times, enable a more complete and comprehensive assessment of the relative outcomes of alternative procedures (including doing nothing). It is still under development and has several features that are in need of further careful thought.[15,16] But it has the singular merit of isolating very clearly most of the key issues that require resolution when one is trying to assess the contribution to 'health' that health care can make. One such issue, for example, concerns how a QALY for one individual is to be compared with a QALY for someone else. Some adopt a position of what I have called 'QALY egalitarianism',[17] viz. a QALY is of equal social value to whomsoever it may accrue and regardless of the QALYs previously enjoyed or in prospect,[18] but this is not inherent in the method, which highlights the need for judgements of this kind without dictating their solution. The method is also useful in identifying the kinds of skills and status that may be appropriate for making the various kinds of judgement embodied in outcome assessment. Some of these are clinical (suggesting that clinicians may be the appropriate persons to be making these judgements) while others are quasi-political judgements (where patients, or potential patients, or their spokespersons such as their personal physicians may be appropriate). Here there is a host of ethical issues for resolution: dimensions in which benefit is to be measured; scaling and measurement; trade-offs between them; trade-offs between beneficiaries. Many of these will be settled in culturally specific ways so that what appears right in one place at one time may not be right elsewhere.

But let it not be thought that these issues are inherent only in this formal approach to outcome measurement. On the contrary, it is easy to see that judgements of this sort are implicit in all resource allocation decisions taken at all levels: for example, a decision to include a particular procedure in an insurance benefits package, a decision to open a new ward (or to close one), a decision to purchase (or not to purchase) the latest imaging technology for a hospital. The fact that the anticipated health benefit is often left implicit, or is proxied by imperfect process or throughput indicators, or is merely asserted without supporting evidence by those whose professional interests are being furthered or damaged, does not mean that implicit judgements about outcome are not being made. The important distinction is not that judgements are or are not being made but rather that they are being made implicitly by people who may or may not be qualified (professionally and ethically) to make them, in a way that is hard to scrutinise, in a way that is hard to assess subsequently in terms of its rightness or wrongness, in contrast to a way that allows the efficiency and ethicality of the decision to be clearly addressed. These other ways may be familiar and comfortable for decision-makers, but these do not seem very powerful arguments for continuing with them. We really need to face up to these uncomfortable implications, not side-step them. It may not be a popular idea that health care resources should be rationed, but that is not really the issue: the issue is how to ration, not whether to ration.

The fourth kind of efficiency is: *providing such a mix of effective services at least resource cost, and on such a scale, that the benefit from having more resources is no larger than their cost*. This is evidently the test for an efficient scale of operation of the health care sector. The additional cost of a QALY (or whatever health outcome measure you prefer) can be expected to rise as increasingly recalcitrant cases are treated, and one should stop putting extra resources into health care when the additional benefit is judged to be no higher than the additional cost. This seems to me to be the appropriate way to think about that vexed question—does the USA spend too much on health care, or does Canada spend too little, as distinct from the sort of question considered previously: has each got the distribution right? It is evidently hugely difficult to judge. But that does not mean that this is not the right and ethical way in which to approach making that judgement. In the final analysis, health care is a means to an end—that of better health. It is not an end in itself. It seems to me to be entirely ethical to enquire as to the benefits and costs generated at existing and alternative imaginable levels of resource commitment with a view to maximising the one relative to the other. But we can only ever do this if the content of 'cost' and 'benefit' are themselves clear and ethically acceptable. Even if, for all sorts of reasons, the system is hard to push towards the level and distribution of resources that we deem to be right, that does not detract from the value of the mental exercise involved in thinking about it in this way, any more than the fact that we each fail to live up to our personal ethical codes is a good reason for not having personal ethical codes. One strives for what is better even when one knows that one will, at least in part, fail. So, I am not necessarily arguing for precise answers but for precise questions. The important thing is to know for what one is striving. Here then are two maxims that I hold dear: *never let the perfect become the enemy of the merely good;* and *our judgements may be imprecise but let us not pretend that the principles are too.* I have argued that 'efficiency' is a value-laden term and that, provided that the objective to be efficiently pursued is itself ethical, then to be efficient is also ethical. It therefore follows that the consideration of an appropriate concept of cost is also ethical. This implication clearly sticks in some gullets, especially, it would seem, clinical gullets. So let us examine this implication in greater detail.

COST

Some years ago Dr Erich Loewy from Glen Falls in New York State wrote to the *New England Journal of Medicine* of his concern at the proliferation of articles with 'cost–benefit' in their titles. His concern was an ethical one and its essence seems to be encapsulated in the following excerpt from his letter: 'Inherent in these articles is the view that choices will be predicated not only on the basis of *strictly clinical considerations* but also on the basis of economic considerations as they may affect the patient, the hospital, and society ... *(S)uch considerations are not germane to ethical medical practice* ... and they serve to orientate physicians towards considerations of economics, which is not their legitimate problem ... A physician who changes his or her way of practising medicine because of cost rather than *purely medical considerations* has indeed embarked on the 'slippery slope' of compromised ethics and waffled priorities'[19] (my italics).

I want for the moment to set aside the implications of this view for the personal relationship between doctor and patient until the next section. Here I want just to explore it at the more macro level of decision-making that I have been considering to this point.

This view may be summarized in the following maxim: 'It is the doctor's duty to do all possible for the patient regardless of cost'. At the macro level of decision-making, one is concerned essentially with questions to do with the amount of resources that should be put at the disposal of physicians (beds, diagnostic equipment, and so on). We may also be concerned with that ultimate resource: the appropriate number of physicians. To claim at this level that cost should not (on ethical grounds) be a factor affecting such decisions made by physicians seems to imply (and I think necessarily does) either that whatever the benefit is perceived to be (does it matter by whom?), so long as it is positive, but no matter how small, the resources ought to be provided; or else that these are decisions properly to be taken by appropriate persons with managerial and/or political responsibility but that it is never appropriate for these decision-makers to be practising physicians. Neither view seems ethically tenable. The former is not tenable because it implicitly elevates health care to an overarching and dominant status above all the other good things of life: a little better health is always worth having whatever it costs in terms of education, leisure activity, good housing, or what you will. There may be some who take such an extreme view, but I doubt if Dr Loewy was one. The second view seems ethically unacceptable because it seems clear that although a medical training does not qualify one to pronounce on all the issues of health policy and health care management, it certainly qualifies one to advise on a great many of them and, in so far as one is speaking on behalf of one's patients, who may otherwise have no immediate voice in such decisions at all, to abrogate responsibility in this fashion is to disenfranchise, at least in part, the very people for whom the whole system exists. Economics (in the sense of taking account of cost) thus seems to be an inherent part of decisions of this kind and, moreover, an essential part if these decisions are to be taken ethically. It does not guarantee an ethical outcome of the decisions, of course. Nor is economics the only consideration. But it is one. In reality the cost of whatever you do with resources is the best of the other things that the resources could have been used for and, unless you are going to argue that all non-health care uses of resources have no ethical claim to consideration (which I cannot conceive of anyone arguing who is not a fanatic), then cost is legitimately there amongst the other considerations. Even more fundamentally, the quotation from Loewy raises the question of what a 'purely medical' decision might be (see also Williams[20] to whom I am indebted for several points in this section). It is plain from my previous discussion of the QALY view of benefit that the issues raised explicitly within that framework are in actuality rather general issues which all assessments or measures of benefit must confront and resolve. It is also clear that many of these issues (indeed, nearly all of them) are by no stretch of the imagination 'purely medical' if by this is meant the kind of skilled judgement in which our medical schools train people. Indeed the entire concept of benefit is so thoroughly imbued with important and controversial issues of value[21] that it is an important question as to who is qualified, and by virtue of what, to make such judgements.

In macro decisions, then, it is scarcely possible, let alone unethical, not to consider cost. Still at the macro level, let us turn briefly to 'need'. I want now to turn to the implications of my postulated starting point for the meaning of 'need'. Although this is commonly and correctly seen often as a question in equity, it also has an important interpretation in discussions of efficiency.

NEED AND EQUITY

The idea of need has had a rough ride from economists, including myself and some colleagues who once wrote '... if it is said that "society needs ..." it is not clear whether what is meant implies that the speaker himself needs it, whether society ought to have it in his opinion, whether a majority of members of society want it. Moreover it is not clear whether it is needed regardless of the social and humanitarian cost to society'.[22] I want to suggest that an appropriate notion of need has to be an instrumental notion—the entity asserted to be needed is needed for something, and that any morally compelling aspect of need derives from this more ultimate end. For example, you might assert that health is needed in order that individuals are enabled to fulfil their potential as free persons and to flourish as members of a community of free persons. In our present context, however, it seems sensible to take health itself as the proximate end and consider the need for health care. If better health is indeed an ethical end of the health care system, then it seems to follow that a need for health care can arise only when a patient has a capacity to benefit from the consumption of health services. This immediately ties the notion of need in with my previous discussion of effectiveness. If the care is not effective, it cannot be said to be needed. If the technology that would improve someone's health for the better does not currently exist, current services cannot be said to be needed (though it may well be that research is needed). In deciding what needs shall be met, however, it is essential to be able to form a judgement about the likely size of the benefit (in terms, say, of enhanced health). So, if needs are to be fairly met (for example, equal treatment for equal need) it becomes important to be able to measure and make informed judgements about capacity to benefit. It is also worth noting that an important element of capacity to benefit is that it must be seen in terms of changes in health status. An absolutely or relatively high mortality or morbidity rate does not in itself indicate a high capacity to benefit: that depends on whether there is a capacity for the rate to be reduced sufficiently by the application of the relevant resources for it to command a priority relative to other needs. Moreover, it is the contribution of health care to the potential health improvement that is important. Many conditions are, for example, self-limiting, so one is concerned with the faster recovery that health care enables rather than the probability of recovery itself. In other cases one may not actually expect a pay-off in terms of better health than before, but rather in terms of better health than would otherwise have been the case—amelioration rather than cure, reduction rather than elimination of disability, slowing rather than stopping deteriorations.

Indeed, one may go further. If positive capacity to benefit is a necessary condition for a need to exist, it is scarcely sufficient, for the need in question is a need for resources. We might for convenience generalise this as a need for particular rates of real expenditure: it is this expenditure that is necessary (viz. needed) if capacity to benefit is to be realised, and it seems natural to consider that a need exists so long as there is a capacity to benefit from additional real expenditure. Someone's need, therefore, in a complete sense, is for whatever real expenditure on effective care will exhaust their capacity to benefit—note, *effective* care. Resources cannot be held to be needed when they are ineffectively deployed. Even equity, in the sense of proportionality between use of resources and need, requires efficiency![23]

A characteristic of this interpretation of need is that it is not absolute. Indeed, it raises all the questions of relative priorities attached to the many components of health that arise when one considers multi-dimensional constructs such as the QALY.

Need, in an efficiency context, focuses on the least cost methods of realising individuals' capacities to benefit, and an efficient allocation of resources is one in which the marginal capacity to benefit in all activities is equalised per dollar of real resources. If the health gain from adding a dollar's expenditure to one type of activity exceeds the health loss from taking that dollar away from another type of activity, the former is more efficient than the latter, and overall health is the greater for making that transfer. Another way of putting this is to require that marginal met need (in dollars) per unit of health gain be everywhere equalised. The equity counterpart is that resources ought to be distributed in proportion to need (equal real expenditure for equal need and proportionately more real expenditure for more need) in all circumstances where the resources available are insufficient to meet all needs—Oregon generalised to the whole health care system! Efficient resource allocation may clash with the equitable allocation, and it is familiar enough that a tradeoff between equity and efficiency may have to be made. This may be uncomfortable, but it is scarcely news. What is also uncomfortable, but perhaps more newsworthy, is that since both efficiency and equity are highly ethical and since equity embodies the cost-effectiveness component of efficiency, it follows that these economic categories of thinking are inherent in doing what is ethically right in allocating health care resources. Their disregard is unethical.

I want now to turn to the more micro ethical level of the individual doctor–patient relationship. A characteristic of the macro approach is that the patient is anonymous or 'statistical'. In making plans at whatever level for the provision of resources for future needs, one is necessarily dealing with populations of imagined patients, who are in a sense 'average' people, about whose needs responsible judgements have to be made, where the necessary value judgements are exercised on behalf of groups, and future groups at that, rather than named individuals with whom the physician has a personal relationship and a personal obligation.

DOCTOR–PATIENT RELATIONSHIPS

Principal–agent theory holds that doctors are (or should be) perfect agents for their patients (the principals), which in a parodied version might be held to require that physicians should be indifferent to all interests other than those of patients, indifferent to the impact of recommendations made for the patient on the doctor's remuneration, indifferent to the demands of the doctor's spouse and family on his or her time, indifferent to the demands of social life on the doctor's time. No sacrifice that can be made will (or should) fail to be made on behalf of the patient. Plainly this is a parody. Doctors do at this micro level take account of cost—at least the cost to them of their own time. They also often feel it right to take account of costs to patients too, whether out of pocket or non-financial (for example, the value of a patient's time). And one cannot say that they are acting unethically or being unfaithful agents in taking such costs into account. But these are costs of just time, and time is just one resource out of many. All costs represent sacrificed opportunities that could have been devoted to the betterment of patients' health or to some other good cause. If, then, it is ethical to take account of the physician's time, why should it be regarded as uniquely special? Other people's time (such as nurses and paramedics, as well as patients), drugs, equipment, the use of beds and other capital, are all resources which, if they are used for one patient are denied to another. Each is costly, just as the doctor's own time is costly. In each case the relevant ethical question has to be 'are the costs worth incurring relative to the expected benefit to this patient?' Every physician has to evaluate these costs and benefits for him- or herself. If this sometimes means that attending to someone's relatively minor, self-limiting, or self-healing problems is postponed or put off indefinitely, then—provided that the more important needs of others are attended to—that seems to be ethically quite acceptable. Consider this example from a British GP with a university practice, who also happens to be editor of the *Journal of Medical Ethics*. He is seeing a patient with severe psychological difficulties and listening to an account of the patient's personal anguish. Suddenly the phone rings—a 55-year-old lecturer with a history of chest pains has collapsed in a lecture room. He excuses himself from the patient before him, being the only GP on duty, in order to attend to the patient outside. Why? He has made a judgement about the allocation of his time between the two patients in need and decided that the cost of temporarily neglecting the one is justified by the greater immediate need of the other. His response, of course, may have been different had the distressed patient in the consulting room been suicidal, or the other patient notably histrionic. But under the circumstances his action, which certainly took account of cost in the only relevant economic sense of that word, which is the value of his time in its next best use, seems entirely ethical and, moreover, consistent with the concept of need that I have outlined above. So the efficiency requirements have been met. All that has changed is that the identities of the two patients were known to the physician, who used this special knowledge to make a decision that was forced on him by circumstances, and to make it in a way that seems on the face of it quite acceptable.

Dr Gillon also tells another instructive tale.[24] A woman with arthritis made an appointment and asked for the latest and most expensive non-steroidal anti-inflammatory drug (NSAID) on the market, about which she had read. Dr Gillon suggested that she start with an ordinary, generally effective, and much cheaper NSAID with no worse side-effects than the other more expensive drug, i.e. aspirin. Dr. Gillon tells us that the patient was outraged. She wanted the best and only the best—and transferred to another GP. Was Gillon acting unethically in this case—withholding, at least in the first instance, the more expensive product and trying something cheaper first? He made, of course, a judgement about unjustified cost. If he had had a limited budget for pharmaceuticals, then the nature of this judgement seems to be much the same as the kind of judgement required in the earlier example when he was concerned with the allocation of his time. He may, of course, have made the wrong decision. It may also be that the resources at his disposal for drug prescriptions were inadequate (and ethically speaking too small as well). But in this case, as in the earlier case, it seemed inherent in his situation that it was inescapably necessary to take account of cost. His drug budget, like his time, was not infinite. Indeed, I suggest that it is in the nature of nearly all clinical decisions that costs are taken into account. Doctors already do it. It is almost second nature to them that they should do. The budgets may bite a bit harder in Canada or the UK than they do for some US client groups where resources are relatively abundant. But this is a question of degree—and in particular of the amount of capacity to benefit that your resources force you not to realise—rather than a question of principle, that is, whether it is right to take costs into account at all.

It is sometimes suggested that the kind of cost–benefit way of thinking about health care resource allocation that is implied by my starting point is appropriate only in macro decisions to do with setting the resource limits within which individual doctors might then be free to exercise their professional discretion 'regardless of cost'. For example, in the case of Dr Gillon's arthritic patient, it was not actually the case that he had a drug budget. Until recently, drug spending by GPs in the UK was open-ended. The obligation felt by Gillon in respect of cost-effective prescribing was in all probability one that he was not as a GP well placed to discharge. After all, his perception of how any savings made as the result of his stewardship would have been used must have been highly imperfect. What if he had believed that the savings would have gone on 'wasteful bureaucracy'? In short, the circumstances of his practice (as with all British GPs at that time) were such as to make the opportunity cost of his actions obscure and therefore his judgement less well informed. The system was not such as to encourage or enable decisions to be made that accorded with our postulated ethical imperative. Or consider a more general case: that of the physician acting as proponent for his or her patients in demanding a larger share of the resources available for health care. While the individual physician may be a good judge of the needs (in my sense of the word) of his or her own patients, he or she will be much less able to evaluate the similar claims of other physicians on behalf of their patients. Resolving this conflict evidently requires the exercise of a macro efficiency/equity judgement that transcends the perceptions of an individual practitioner. So it is important to get these things institutionally right in the sense of clarity as to the extent of the doctor's discretion, and economically right in the sense of giving him or her the right bundle of resources within which to exercise micro discretion. But it is also clear that, even if these things have been got right, it is still not true that a 'two-tier' approach to cost works: in which the cost–benefit judgements are applied only to the macro budget-setting decision, while the individual clinical judgement can be made solely on benefit judgements concerning the patient who happens to be there. The reason is obvious: the resources put at the physician's disposal (including his or her time) still have valued alternative uses within the range of demands that are put upon them in the context of a particular medical practice. These alternatives forgone are costs, and the only difference between the macro decision and the more personal micro decision is that the identity of the gainers and the losers is known. This may raise all sorts of questions which I am not competent to deal with, to do with the degree to which patients are given reasons for decisions and advice, or to do with sharing with patients the difficulties presented by limited resources, but one thing they do not banish is the necessity to take account of cost. The doctor may pretend to patients that he or she does not take it into account, and may even deceive himself or herself into believing that he or she does not take it into account. Indeed it may even be crucially important in dealing with patients to cherish the illusion that costs do not come into judgement about what is to be done. If, however, to be sure that what is being done really is ethical, then the balance of cost and benefit must be examined in everything. In short, not to take account of cost is what is unethical: quite the contrary to what the 'regardless of cost' school of medical thought would have us believe.

Let us move away from cost and consider another question that brings us to the heart of the doctor–patient relationship and relates to the way in which a named individual's values (and hence benefits and needs) are taken into account in medical decision-making.[25] Consider the following common version of the ethical duty of a doctor acting as a perfect agent for the patients in his or her care:

The *doctor* is there to give the *patient* all the information the *patient* needs in order that the *patient* can make a decision; the *doctor* should implement that decision once the *patient* has made it. Here you see two roles carefully distinguished: that of the *adviser*, respecting the individuality and preferences of the—presumed rational—client; and that of the professional *responder* to demand, providing the appropriate care demanded. But now delete all the words in italics, and reverse them. This is now what we get:

The *patient* is there to give the *doctor* all the information the *doctor* needs in order that the *doctor* can make a decision; the *patient* should implement that decision once the *doctor* has made it.

That looks a bit different—and perhaps more familiar? It reverses the nature of 'compliance' for one thing. It also puts the patient firmly in his or her place. There is the clear danger in this version that the autonomy of the patient is compromised, that he or she becomes 'objectified', and that the doctor is master and the patient servant. It may usually be that the doctor has a better knowledge of what, for the sake of a convenient shorthand, we might call 'technical matters'. This is an asymmetry in the doctor–patient relationship. The second version raises a second kind of asymmetry in the doctor–patient relationship. It is also usually the case that the patient has a better knowledge of his or her own preferences, for example in willingness to accept risks. One person may prefer laryngectomy and a 60% chance of a 3-year survival for cancer of the vocal chords, while another may prefer radiation to spare the voice at the cost of a lower chance of surviving 3 years. Here is another issue of value which can hardly be held to be 'purely medical'. This second version of the agency relationship thus raises the question, which is largely empirical rather than ethical, of the efficiency with which information about preferences can be conveyed from patient to doctor. In principle, the outcome would appear to be the same whether the doctor conveyed (all) the known (to him or her) information on 'technical matters' for the patient to decide; or the patient conveyed (all) the preference information for the doctor to decide. In practice, the balance between the two versions will probably depend on a meta-judgement by the doctor about his or her ability to extract and convey information and on his or her ability to communicate effectively with the patient, which may take time, several consultations, consultations with professional people other than the doctor in question (e.g. other doctors, nurses), and consultations with the patient's family. So this is a third kind of asymmetry, which may go either way: an asymmetry in communication skills.

WHO IS THE PATIENT?

But who is the patient? I have so far treated this question as if it were answered implicitly by 'the one in front of the doctor'. A doctor clearly has responsibility for current patients, but what about those waiting to be seen? What about those known to be in need but who have failed, for whatever reason, to make contact? What about the general public, any one of whom may come to be in need at some time? Has the doctor no ethical responsibility for these? Most doctors would affirm, I conjecture, that there is such a responsibility. But how, then, should such a responsibility be discharged? In the case of unmet need, if it is ethical for a doctor to ignore the manner in which the patient before him or her gets to be there (the only thing mattering being that the patient is actually there), then one is saying (amongst other things) that one is indifferent between the plight of the insured and the uninsured, those able to pay and those unable to pay, those living near the practice who find it easy to get there and those more distant, those who are well enough informed (or hypochondriacal enough) to get themselves along by hook or by crook and those less well informed or complacent. The ethicality of that hardly stands scrutiny. So, if it is unethical to ignore the process that has brought the patient before the doctor, it is ethical to take account of it. Such considerations must form a part of judgements as to what it means to have an efficient health care system, granted that needs are to be efficiently met in the pursuit of our postulated health objective. These judgements cannot be made by considering only the 'purely medical', at least not if by 'purely medical' one means to exclude cost and supposes that benefit can be judged without reference to the quality of life of patients, current and future.

I conclude from all this that the ethical practitioner making either macro or micro medical decisions has to be an economist! Not, of course, in the professionally qualified sense and certainly not in any crude financial accounting sense, but in the more fundamental sense that one's judgement needs constantly to be exercised by questions like: is the health benefit I predict from this course of action more or less than that from an alternative? Is the benefit worth the expected cost? How much do I actually know about the benefit and how well does it reflect my patient's values? How reliable is my diagnosis and prognosis? Am I on top of the available evidence on effectiveness in the literature? How accurate is my perception of cost? After all, what could be more ethical than to seek to ensure—as economists are always urging—that the only things worth doing are those for which the benefit outweighs the cost? I am not pretending that these judgements are easy, especially when you are making them as an agent on behalf of someone—probably a very distressed someone—who is dependent on you. Behaving in an upright and ethical way never is easy! But I do assert that it cannot be ethical to ignore cost and to take a cavalier attitude to the vital value questions thrown up by the practice of medicine. I also assert that it cannot be ethical to be inefficient. Again, our judgements about these matters may in practice be imprecise, but let us not pretend that the principles are.

CONCLUSIONS

I have tried to explore some of the implications of the view that a properly ethical objective of the health care system is to maximise the community's health. I am well aware, of course, that 'health' (however you define it) is not the only purpose or product of health services and it does not follow from this view that important dimensions of performance like the supply of information and reassurance, or that comfort, courtesy, respect for individual dignity, turning up for appointments on time, and so on, are beyond its ken, nor that the hotel dimensions of institutional care are unimportant. Process is important, as well as outcome, and if each is a good, it is ethically incumbent on us to be efficient here as well as in the matters on which I have been concentrating, and for the same ethical reasons. It also seems likely, however, that equity considerations, in contrast to efficiency considerations, may lead us to apply different equity criteria to at least some of these from those applied, say, to meeting needs for health care. For example, if you follow the Aristotelian tradition, you may take the view that equal needs for health care demand equal treatment. I conjecture that many holding that view would not, however, also subscribe to the view that persons who are equal in that respect should necessarily be forced to consume the same style of hotel services. After all, we do not seem to require it in the hotel sector proper of the economy; why require it in the hospital-as-a-hotel?

My purpose has been to try to show that the set of considerations embodied in the use of the term 'efficiency' can be seen as highly ethical—but only as ethical as the objective which is sought efficiently to be attained. I have also tried to show that, granted this end, it is unethical for medical decision-making to ignore costs—costs in the core meaning of that word as 'valued forgone opportunities for using resources', and that this is the case not only at the system design level, but also at the macro level of anonymous or 'statistical' patients and at the personal micro level of the doctor–patient relationship. I also suggested a meaning for that controversial and much misused word 'need' which is both operational and, more importantly in the present context, consistent with the ethical starting point of my discussion. I have tried to show that the issues embodied in the notion of 'benefit' from health care are complex and subtle and that their solution at the macro level may be rather different from their solution at the micro level—but that at neither level is it sufficient to treat benefit as a 'purely medical' consideration. I have also tried to show that economic efficiency is also inherent in at least one common approach to equity, that is, allocation of resources in proportion to need. 'Cost' is thus all-pervasive.

The UK, Canada and the USA have a long way to go in creating a health care system that encourages a truly ethical practice of medicine. We shall never fully get there, of course, whatever our systems. But that does not mean that we can do without a gold standard to tell us how far short of the ideal we may be falling and to inform us about changes in the structure of the system, and the way in which the professionals within it work, that may push us in the right direction. Ethical principles do not become unimportant because we cannot live up to them. They are important precisely because we know we never can.

REFERENCES

1. Donabedian, A. Social responsibility for personal health services: an examination of basic values. *Inquiry* 1971; **8**: 3–19.
2. Tobin, J. On limiting the domain of inequality. *Journal of Law and Economics* 1970; **13**: 263–278.
3. Culyer, A. J., Maynard, A. K. M. and Williams, A. H. Alternative systems of health care provision: an essay on motes and beams. In: M. Olsen (ed.) *A new approach to the economics of health care*, Washington, American Enterprise Institute (1981).
4. Culyer, A. J. The promise of a reformed NHS: an economist's angle. *British Medical Journal*. 1991; **302**: 1253–1256.
5. Cochrane, A. L. Effectiveness and efficiency: random reflections on health services, London, Nuffield Provincial Hospitals Trust, 1972.
6. Glantz, S. A. Biostatistics: how to detect, correct and prevent errors in the medical literature. *Circulation* 1980; **61**: 1–7.
7. McPherson, K. International differences in medical care practices. *Health Care Financing Review* 1989; Annual Supplement, 9–20.
8. Rachlis, M. and Kushner, C. Second opinion: what's wrong with Canada's health care system and how to fix it. Toronto, Harper and Collins, 1989.
9. Sackett, D. L. Evaluation of health services. In: J. M. Last (ed.) Maxcy-Rosenau public health and preventive medicine (11th edn), New York, Appleton-Century-Crofts, 1980.
10. Sheehan, T. J. The medical literature—let the reader beware. *Archives of Internal Medicine* 1980; **140**: 472–474.
11. Wennberg, J. and Gittelsohn, A. Variations in medical care among small areas. *Scientific American*. 1982; **246**: 100–111.
12. McKeown, T. *The Modern Rise of Population*. London, Arnold, 1976.

13. McPherson, K., Wennberg, J., Hovind, O. and Clifford, P. Small area variations in the use of common surgical procedures: an international comparison of New England, England and Norway. *New England Journal of Medicine* 1982; **307**: 1310–1314.
14. Torrance, G. W. Measurement of health state utilities for economic appraisal. *Journal of Health Economics* 1986; **5**: 1–30.
15. Loomes, G. and McKenzie, L. The scope and limitations of QALY measures. In: S. Baldwin, C. Godfrey and C. Propper (eds) *Quality of Life: Perspectives and Policies*. London, Routledge, 1990.
16. Mehrez, A. and Gafni, A. Quality-adjusted-life-years, utility theory, and healthy years equivalents. *Medical Decision Making* 1989; **9**: 141–154.
17. Culyer, A. J. Conflicts between equity concepts and efficiency in health: a diagrammatic approach. *Osaka Economic Papers* 1991; **40**: 141–154.
18. Williams, A. H. Economics of coronary artery bypass grafting. *British Medical Journal* 1985; **291**: 326–329.
19. Loewy, E. H. Cost should not be a factor in medical care. *New England Journal of Medicine*. 1980; **302**: 697.
20. Williams, A. H. Medical ethics: health service efficiency and clinical freedom, Folio 2, Nuffield/York Portfolios, London, Nuffield Provincial Hospitals Trust, 1980.
21. Culyer, A. J. Need, values and health status measurement. In: A. J. Culyer and K. G. Wright (eds) *Economic Aspects of Health Services*, London, Martin Robertson, 1978, 9–31.
22. Culyer, A. J., Lavers, R. J. and Williams, A. H. Social Indicators: health. *Social Indicators* 1971; **2**: 31–42.
23. Culyer, A. J. and Wagstaff, A. Need, equality and social justice. Discussion Paper 90, York, Centre for Health Economics, 1992.
24. Gillon, R., Ethics, economics and general practice. In: G. Mooney and A. Mcguire (eds) *Medical Ethics and Economics in Health Care*, Oxford, Oxford University Press, 1988, 114–134.
25. Williams, A. H. Ethics, clinical freedom and the doctor's role. In: A. J. Culyer, A. K. Maynard and J. Posnett (eds) *Competition in Health Care: Reforming the NHS*, London, Macmillan, 1990, 178–191.

CHAPTER 2

The Canadian health care system: a model for America to emulate?

C. David Naylor
Sunnybrook Health Science Centre, and the Institute for Clinical Evaluative Sciences in Ontario, Toronto, Ontario, Canada.

INTRODUCTION

The American health care system is under pressure to adopt reforms that will improve patient access and allow more equitable delivery of essential medical and hospital services. The recent election of Bill Clinton as President has made reform a certainty. However, while various opinion polls suggest that a majority of Americans favour some form of national health insurance (NHI) plan,[1,2] there is no consensus on the direction that a new American plan should take. Canada's federal–provincial system of universal health insurance is frequently held up as a potential model for emulation, and support for moving towards a Canadian-style system has been offered by senior citizens' lobby groups, public hospital associations, and prominent medical organisations such as the American College of Physicians.[3] On the other hand, a more limited set of reforms has been endorsed by both organised labour and

North American Health Care Policy in the 1990s
Edited by A. King, T. Hyclak, S. McMahon and R. Thornton

industrial leaders, with a Canadian-style system explicitly rejected by the insurance industry, conservative political groups, and the American Medical Association (AMA). Indeed, in 1989 the AMA launched a $2.5 million advertising campaign to warn Americans of the hazards of following Canada's lead.[4]

Data presented below suggest, on balance, that America would benefit from NHI patterned in part after Canada's plan. But while Canada's Medicare system embodies admirable principles and can claim conspicuous successes, the Canadian model has many problems in common with the American approach, along with its own unique drawbacks. This chapter accordingly offers an overview of the Canadian health care system, draws some comparisons with the American scene, and points out strengths and weaknesses of the Canadian approach.

Before proceeding, it should be noted that the Canadian system is a federal–provincial programme, with ten component provincial plans that differ somewhat from each other. The province of Ontario will serve as the principal source for Canadian data, because of its size (9.7 million, with more than a third of the nation's population and medical facilities), and the author's familiarity with its system. However, information about other provinces will be introduced as appropriate.

POLITICAL CONTEXT

The obvious cultural and political similarities between Canada and the USA make it more attractive for Americans to consider importation of the Canadian approach to health care. Despite those similarities, there are important differences in the political values and institutions of Canada and the USA.[5,6] With a small population (now about 27 million) spread over an enormous surface area, Canada has long relied on an interventionist federal government for nation-building. Government involvement in the economy has been prominent for a century. Political ideologies also differ. Socialist governments have held power in four provinces, and currently govern Ontario. American themes of libertarianism and individualism are muted in Canada, where many public sector initiatives and social programmes were actually launched by the Conservative Party. Furthermore, in each province and at the federal level, Canadian governments operate under a parliamentary system which imposes caucus discipline and reduces the influence of interest groups.[7]

As William L. Roper has noted in a comment on NHI from the White House staff perspective,[8] America's complex system of checks and balances makes it far more difficult to initiate sweeping reforms in health care. Among other features of the American political scene that militate against the development of a political consensus and action plan for NHI are: the sheer size and diversity of the USA, ideological antipathy to government intervention in the economy, turn-over of high-ranking civil servants in the executive branch of government, and the strong role of interest groups in electoral politics.

One pertinent similarity is that both Canada and the USA are federal entities, with constitutionally determined divisions in powers. As will be reviewed below, in Canada this has allowed provincial governments to act as beach-heads for health reform initiatives. A parallel trend is belatedly emerging in America, as states such as Hawaii, Minnesota and Oregon move ahead with distinctive approaches to the problem of providing coverage.[9,10] A recurrent problem in Canada has been disproportionate federal taxing authority when administrative responsibility for most social and educational programmes lies with the provinces. Conflict over the fiscal terms of Canadian federal programmes is therefore inevitable, and parallel conflicts have latterly emerged in America as the states shoulder a growing fiscal burden from national health programmes, most notably Medicaid. However, NHI in Canada was introduced before the recent debt crisis, and was made possible in part by the ability of the federal government to offer cost-sharing provisions that no province could reject. At present, the federal government in Canada points to the national debt in explaining its reduced support for provincially administered health and social programmes—a trend that could have profound implications for the future of Canadian health care (see below).

THE CANADIAN SYSTEM: EVOLUTION TO UNIVERSALITY

Understanding Canada's health insurance programme requires some appreciation of its historical antecedents.[7,11] Early general hospitals were variously established through religious or capitalist philanthropy, or by direct government intervention. Municipal levies eventually supported the operations of most hospitals, but contributions of provincial funds seldom occurred until the Great Depression of the 1930s caused general financial hardships. From then on, per diems for so-called indigent patients were increasingly provided by provincial rather than local arrangements. The Depression also proved a catalyst for the growth of non-profit private hospital insurance sponsored by provincial hospital associations—Canada's equivalent of the Blue Cross plans.[7,11,12] However, no province had instituted a universal hospital insurance plan until Saskatchewan's first socialist government did so in 1947.[9,13] Other provinces gradually followed suit.

As to medical services, the marketplace in Canada differed sharply from that which developed in many European countries. For example, in Britain there was a division between general practitioners (GPs) and specialists, rooted in the guild antecedents of both groups. British GPs, who served primarily the working and lower middle classes, were frequently forced into so-called lodge practice, working on a capitation or even fixed retainer basis for consumer groups. But in Canada, as in the USA, lodge practice never took hold enough to create momentum for alternatives to fee-for-service practice. Salaried and capitated primary care practices were limited largely to remote areas, e.g. under Saskatchewan's famed Municipal Doctor plans, in mining towns, and in similar industrial situations.[7] The 1930s brought severe financial hardship to the

Canadian medical profession, and led organised medicine to press, at both federal and provincial levels, for first-dollar government-sponsored health insurance for low-income persons and the unemployed.[7,14] A number of provinces eventually did institute plans for payment of doctors serving the destitute and unemployed—a movement parallel to the earlier changes in the public hospital sector.

Through the 1930s and 1940s, organised medicine also established increasing numbers of medically sponsored prepayment plans, generally offering first-dollar coverage and providing direct payment from plan to practitioner.[7,11,12] These plans paved the way for the eventual institution of the current Medicare programme. Four motives can be identified from analysis of the voluntary prepayment movement under organised medical auspices: (i) to ensure financial security for doctors and reduce the role of direct financial dealings in doctor–patient interactions; (ii) to meet consumers' desires for insurance against the rising costs of illness, as medical practice became somewhat more technology intensive; (iii) to head off the threat of salaried prepaid practice plans and community clinics; and (iv) to forestall intervention by private for-profit insurance agencies that were seen as potential threats to professional autonomy even in the 1940s.[7] Opposition to government intervention was not a major motivation in these early developments; indeed, medical leaders highlighted the concept that the plans could serve as a model for the broader-ranging government programmes that were widely viewed as desirable and inevitable.[7]

Thus, prior to the late 1950s, Canada's health care prepayment system included a complex amalgam of public and private plans—provincial medical and hospital coverage for recipients of social assistance, universal hospital insurance programmes in a few provinces, private medical and hospital insurance on a non-profit basis sponsored by provider organisations, and a limited amount of market share held by investor-owned insurers. A national programme of first-dollar coverage for hospital care and related diagnostic services was legislated in 1957–58, with implementation during the Conservative government of the prairie populist, John Diefenbaker. Federal cost-sharing for provincial hospital insurance allowed the socialist government in Saskatchewan to expand its programme to the physician sector, and the first universal medical services plan was implemented there in 1962. By this time, organised medicine had become more conservative, and its policy was that governments should limit themselves to mandating and subsidising enrolment in existing private plans. The Saskatchewan plan sparked an intense dispute and a 3-week doctors' strike.[7,11,15] However, a subsequent Royal Commission into national medical insurance, chaired by Mr Justice Emmett Hall,[16] led to a strong endorsement of a Medicare plan on the lines of the one now operative. In 1968, the federal framework for a national medical insurance plan was set in place, with transfers of tax dollars to provinces offering programmes that met federal conditions; all provinces and northern territories were participating fully by 1971.

Although the term Medicare should, strictly speaking, be reserved for the medical services component of the federal–provincial health insurance system, it is now used generically for the combined medical and hospital insurance programmes. The early years of the combined medical and hospital programme were remarkable for their success. The economy was reasonably buoyant, and governments were able to afford the programme without either major tax increases or indebtedness. Medical practitioners enjoyed unprecedented incomes, pushed up by three forces: fee schedule increases adopted by medical associations in several provinces to cushion their members against collective bargaining that would start after institution of universal government-administered prepayment; a rise in per capita utilisation of services following Medicare; and the elimination of bad debts with all patients fully insured. Hospitals, too, were expanding. Growth in the gross national product (GNP) was such that despite the major increases in expenditures on health services, the sector's share of GNP did not increase during most of the 1970s.

As the 1970s continued, however, inflationary pressures led provincial governments to take an increasingly hard line in collective bargaining with organised medicine. General wage and price controls were eventually implemented as an inflation-fighting measure. Meanwhile, medical school output continued unchecked, with a major growth in physician supply across Canada. The result, not surprisingly, was a striking erosion of real medical incomes.

The original Medicare legislation in every province but Quebec had allowed practitioners the latitude to make extra charges to patients above the negotiated fee schedule*. During the late 1970s the number of practitioners making these extra charges in provinces other than Quebec increased greatly, and led to widespread concern that the principles of Medicare were being eroded.[17] In 1980, Mr Justice Emmett Hall was summoned from retirement by the federal government to review this situation. Hall recommended national adoption of the Quebec approach: if a doctor stayed in the Medicare plan, he or she would have to accept the negotiated tariff as full payment without making extra charges to patients. If a doctor wanted to charge more, his or her patients would have to pay all charges without any right to reimbursement. The result would be enormous pressure on practitioners to stay within the Medicare plan. However, to protect the profession from the lopsided monopsony situation such fiscal arrangements created, Hall endorsed binding arbitration as a means of settling all fee schedule disputes.[18]

The provinces were not enthused about Hall's proposals, and the federal government was uncertain how to proceed. Finally in 1984 the federal government passed the Canada Health Act.[19] This legislation imposed dollar-for-dollar reductions in federal transfer payments to provinces that allowed hospitals to levy user fees or doctors to make charges to patients above and beyond negotiated tariffs. Within 2 years, all provinces passed legislation to abolish additional charges for

---

* In Quebec, the law as passed in 1970 did not allow patients to be reimbursed upon presenting bills for publicly insured services. Doctors were therefore forced either to bill the plan directly, or to convince patients that paying in full outside the plan was worthwhile.

publicly insured services. Organised medicine unsuccessfully protested the federal and provincial laws; the protest in Ontario included a protracted campaign of service interruptions.[19,20]

CURRENT ADMINISTRATIVE FEATURES

Where, then, do matters stand in early 1993? Each of the ten provincial plans is universal, offers coverage that is portable across the country, is publicly administered on a non-profit basis by a single agency of the Ministry of Health, and pays fully for most medical and hospital services. Long-term care is also universally insured.[21] Coverage for semi-private or private hospital rooms can be purchased through Blue Cross plans, but private insurance is generally prohibited for publicly insured services. Indeed, the public monopoly provisions of the Canadian health insurance legislation are more stringent than virtually any in Europe. Provinces vary, but most offer only limited public coverage for services not provided by physicians. For example, dental coverage commonly includes only inpatient surgery, while optometric coverage is limited to refractions and partial payment for corrective lenses. Outpatient prescription medications are publicly insured only for senior citizens, those in receipt of social welfare benefits, and persons with certain communicable and/or chronic diseases where special provisions have been made.

For publicly insured services, the predominant source of funding is taxation. Premiums have generally been phased out altogether or transformed into employer health taxes. About 75% of all health service expenditures flow through the public sector. This is typical for countries in the Organization for Economic Cooperation and Development; the USA is exceptional in that under 45% of expenditures are in the public sector.[22] Canadian private expenditures include private insurance and out-of-pocket charges for services that are outside the universal public plans, particularly outpatient prescriptions, routine dental care, and various other services noted above.

Most Canadian physicians remain in private practice, and fee-per-item of service is the dominant mode of remuneration. In some specialties, means around the ban on extra-billing have been developed, consisting largely in extra charges for services that might be considered routine, but are not expressly described in the benefits schedule (e.g. telephone consultations, letters for employers, photocopying of records) and can therefore be categorised as 'uninsured'. The sums involved range from trivial to substantial, and governments have generally turned a blind eye to this entrepreneurship.

Despite enthusiasm on the part of health ministries, there has been only limited experimentation with alternative funding arrangements, and even this has occurred almost exclusively in the primary care as opposed to specialist sector. For example, in Ontario, 95% of the population receives its primary care from the fee-for-service sector, and of the remainder most are served by private practitioners who have simply elected a group capitation payment. In early 1991 there were about 70 such groups, called health service organisations, with 300 000 patients and about 400 family physicians enrolled. Only 1% of Ontarians are served by salaried GPs in about 30 community health centres run by boards of local trustees.[23] In Quebec a deliberate attempt was made to blanket the province with such primary care centres. The 158 *centres locaux de santé communautaires* in Quebec aim to integrate health and social services and are similar to Ontario's community health centres, but fee-for-service primary care remains dominant. Other provinces are similar to Ontario.[24] Little scientific research has been done comparing the performance of these different primary care models,[25] and extant data are conflicting. For example, an early Quebec study showed community health centres to be more attuned to disease prevention and health promotion;[26] a recent Ontario study found few differences between fee-for-service practice and alternative primary care programmes.[27]

Global increases across the fee schedule are negotiated between each provincial government and medical association; specific allocation of increments generally occurs internally by brokerage among primary care and specialty groups.

Negotiations have frequently been acrimonious, with occasional withdrawal of non-essential medical services during disputes and unilateral imposition of settlements by provincial governments. To consolidate their bargaining positions and avoid the need for strike action, provincial medical bodies have latterly pressed for mandatory payment of annual dues by all private practitioners, along with binding arbitration to settle fee disputes. The latter system is now operative in Manitoba and Ontario.

Hospitals in the acute care sector are all public, in the sense that they are state-dependent contractors and their managers must answer in part to the health ministry. However, because of their origins, the hospitals are actually private, voluntary non-profit corporations. They are run by professional administrators, reporting to community trustees. Each hospital receives a global annual allocation of funds from the province; the global budgets are increased annually, according to the fiscal situation of the government and rather *ad hoc* perceptions of adequacy of hospital services. Supplemental funding is provided for capital renewal and specialised programmes. The latter has allowed government to use fiscal levers to encourage regionalisation of some services, such as open heart surgery, organ transplantation, nuclear magnetic resonance imaging, and so on. Apart from these high-profile and high-cost items where the need for add-on government funding forces rationalisation, inter-institutional coordination has been minimal with little accountability to district or regional planning bodies. Duplication of services remains commonplace, as each hospital tries to be 'all things to all people'. However, severe budgetary pressures in the last 3 years have catalysed some voluntary regional planning, as hospitals try to streamline their operations. Two provinces have moved towards regional restructuring of services, and there is ongoing debate about the merits of putting hospital budgetary management in the hands of regional authorities.

The evolution of Canadian hospitals is in contrast to the American scene. In Canada, universal hospital services prepayment means that all general hospitals are effectively public institutions. In the USA, the passage of Medicare and Medicaid arguably accelerated the movement away from public hospitals by covering a substantial proportion of the population in a fashion that eliminated 'charity care'. Between 1960 and 1980 the number of public hospital beds in America actually shrank by 38% while private beds increased by 61%. Unfortunately, with the erosion of Medicaid, the proportion of persons with low incomes left uncovered has greatly increased over the last decade and thereby created a situation in which a diminished public hospital sector must provide charitable inpatient services for a growing number of uninsured persons.

Canadian hospital occupancy rates typically run 80–85%, as compared to the American average of just over 60% (although the latter figure must be tempered by an appreciation of the public–private division in American hospital beds).[28] For years, Canadian hospitals with operating deficits were given supplemental funds, while those with surpluses were asked to return them. Most provinces have abandoned this system of perverse incentives. For example, in 1987–88 72 of Ontario's 225 hospitals operated at a deficit; no 'bail-out' was provided. Continuing fiscal pressures in the Ontario hospital system have led to widespread downsizing. For the last five complete data years (1987–1991), the hospital days per 1000 population dropped from 1117 to 896, day surgery rose from 53% to 66% of all surgical procedures, and average length of stay fell from 8.7 days to 7.5 days (personal communication: health system management group of the Ontario Ministry of Health). Moreover, American phenomena such as patient 'dumping'[29,30] or hospital insolvency due to unremunerated care are unknown.

HEALTH CARE EXPENDITURES: CANADIAN–AMERICAN COMPARISONS

As shown in Table 2.1, total health expenditures as a percentage of GNP are lower in Canada.[31] By this yardstick,

Table 2.1 System-wide expenditure comparisons as percentage of GNP

	Canada (%)	USA (%)
1971	7.4	7.6
1981	7.7	9.2
1988	8.6	11.5

Source: Adapted from Evans *et al.*, *New England Journal of Medicine* 1989; **320**: 571–577.

Canadian expenditures are comparable to Germany, France, Sweden and the Netherlands.[32] The widening gap between Canada and the USA is attributable in part to faster GNP growth in Canada, leading to relative reduction in proportionate health expenditures. However, a logical fallacy in highlighting Canadian GNP growth is the fact that health expenditures in the USA have grown faster than per capita income, whereas the converse is true in Canada. Thus, if American GNP growth were the same as Canada's, the per capita expenditure differential—discussed below—would be even greater.

Use of the crude GNP as a denominator for such calculations may overstate the differences, since various adjustments to any GNP figure may be defensible.[33] One alternative is to track undeflated or nominal medical expenditure growth in the two countries. This shows parallel increases of about 225% in total health expenditures over the decade 1975–1985.[34] In fact, for the period 1970–1989 the UK actually had the highest growth in nominal per capita expenditure on health care, with Canada slightly outstripping the USA.[32] Adjusting for health care inflation again puts Canada well behind the USA in rate of growth of expenditures on health services. However, this adjustment seems especially problematic, since containing health sectoral inflation and overall expenditures relative to other sectors of the economy is presumably a desirable outcome. One is thus drawn back to measures that compare overall economic growth to nominal health sectoral expenditures. Apart from simple health-to-GNP ratios as presented above, another useful index of this nature is the *rate* of growth in health expenditures relative to per capita GNP.[32] Again Canada did substantially better than the USA for the overall period 1970–1989 (health expenditures growing 10% faster than per capita GNP in Canada, and 30% faster in the USA), but a sagging Canadian economy and deterioration in cost containment brought the two nations into closer proximity in the last decade.

The bottom line is straightforward: Canada and the USA have the two most expensive health care systems in the world in per capita terms, but the 1989 per capita costs were about US $670 in favour of Canada—$2354 in the USA versus $1683 across Canada.[32] These per capita costs are compared to other nations in Table 2.2.

Lower costs in Canada are almost paradoxical. There are no direct financial barriers to care in Canada, and virtually no uninsured persons, in contrast to a substantial minority of uninsured Americans that is estimated between 31 and

Table 2.2 Comparisons of per capita expenditures in US dollars, 1989

Australia	1032
Canada	1683
France	1274
Germany	1232
Italy	1050
Japan	1035
Netherlands	1135
Sweden	1361
UK	836
USA	2354

Source: Adapted from Schieber and Poullier, *Health Affairs* 1991; **10**: 106–116.

37 million persons, with another 50 million deemed financially vulnerable due to inadequate coverage.[3] Actual patient encounters per capita are 55% higher in Canada than in the USA, with 1985 estimates at 8.2 encounters per person in Ontario versus 5.3 per person in the USA (personal communication: D. Weinkauf, director of economics, Ontario Medical Association)—numbers that argue against claims that Canadians suffer from widespread under-provision of medical services due to NHI!

How can lower costs in Canada be explained? At the outset, note that higher numbers of physician claims per patient need not translate to higher medical service costs, since the types and prices of services vary between the two systems. The general explanation for cost containment in Canada is the single-tap theory: whereas the American system flows money to health care through a plethora of variably regulated private and public sources, most Canadian expenditures flow through the provincial health ministries. The provinces can contain growth in hospital budgets by capping annual global increases and similarly limit medical fee increases, leaving number and mix of services per capita as the uncontrolled variables in physician-related expenditures. Not surprisingly, several provinces have also moved to limit fiscal exposure for increasing numbers of mix of services by capping total allowable increases in expenditures, and pro-rating payments to physicians accordingly.

In support of the single-tap theory is the experience in Hawaii, where since 1974 all employers have been obliged to provide employees with a comprehensive package of health insurance benefits. The market is totally dominated by two insurers—Blue Cross and Kaiser Permanente—and costs per capita have been contained at Canadian levels.[9] However, the single-tap explanation does leave open the question of exactly how and where the savings truly occur. Cost differences for three main expenditure areas are shown in Table 2.3 as a percentage of GNP.[31] Major savings on overheads are explicable by administrative economies from having one major prepayment agency in each province. Prospective payments of lump

Table 2.3 Components of expenditure differentials as a percentage of GNP

	Canada	USA
Overheads	0.11	0.59
Hospitals	3.48	4.18
Doctors	1.35	2.07

Source: Evans *et al.*, *New England Journal of Medicine* 1989; **320**: 571–577.

sums to hospitals obviate the need for the ministry to track and pay individual accounts. Physician billings are received as batches of computer cards or actual diskettes, and settled by lump sum payments, again greatly reducing administrative costs. Ironically, half of Canadian physicians surveyed in 1986 believed that overheads would be lower with a private system.[35]

Apart from these direct savings on prepayment administration, similar mechanisms allow hospitals and medical doctors to reduce their overheads, yielding indirect savings (see below). One estimate of the potential savings to America from these three sources of overhead costs[36] can be projected to almost US $50 billion in current dollars. An updated analysis by the same authors documents deteriorating administrative efficiency, and puts the savings from adopting a Canadian-style system even higher, at US $70–80 billion for 1987.[37] Those dollars alone would basically eliminate America's problems with uninsured and underinsured persons. However, such hypothetical savings assume immediate and costless transformation of the American system, when there would be short-term economic dislocation from administrative streamlining.

Cost differences in the hospital sector—which are variously estimated at 20–30% per capita—are not due to overall utilisation. For example, bed utilisation among the elderly has been stable in Canada, but falling rapidly in America. While admission rates are similar, Canada uses almost twice as many general hospital days for its senior citizens due to its greater length of stay. However, American per diem expenditures for the elderly are almost three times higher than in Canada, more than cancelling out the savings from reduced length of stay.[38] Costs per diem in America are only partly due to higher hospital overheads (for reasons noted above). The major difference is a more service-intensive hospitalisation pattern in the USA—more done to each patient per day. In contrast, Canadians have a longer 'tail' on their admissions, consisting in lower-intensity recuperative days after initial diagnosis and treatment.

As shown in Table 2.4, lower intensity per hospital admission in Canada may be due in part to reduced rates of surgical and other procedures. Of interest, a comparison confined to the elderly shows similar rates of pacemaker procedures and valve repairs or replacements, but much greater differences in surgical rates for a more discretionary procedure—coronary bypass surgery.[39] Exceptions such as tonsillectomy notwithstanding, the lower rates of more discretionary surgery in part

Table 2.4 Some annual surgical rates per 100 000 persons in Ontario and the USA, 1985–86

	USA	Ontario
Caesarean section	370	280
Hysterectomy	280	220
Cholecystectomy	200	220
Tonsillectomy	120	270
Oophorectomy/Salpingo-oophorectomy	220	60
Appendectomy	110	110
Prostatectomy	130	160
Coronary surgery	100	40

Source: Compiled by Mr Darrel Weinkauf, Department of Economics, Ontario Medical Association, from the American College of Surgeons' *Socioeconomic Factbook for Surgery, 1987*, and from a 3-month service data set from the Ontario Health Insurance Plan (drawn from billings received between January 1 and June 30, 1986). Adapted from Detsky *et al., Canadian Medical Association Journal* 1990; **142**: 565–572.

reflect the comparatively conservative nature of Canadian medical culture (which overtly styles itself as halfway between American zeal and British conservatism). Rate differentials may also be due to funding constraints that either cap procedural throughput causing pent-up demand to be manifested in waiting lists, or influence providers to accept a more restrained pattern of practice as the norm. However, a 10% increase in capacity was enough to clear away a major problem with open-heart surgery waiting lists in Ontario,[40] even though open-heart surgery rates are more than twice as high in the USA. It therefore appears likely that rate differentials reflect practice styles, rather than funding constraints alone.

The superior cost containment in the Canadian hospital sector has been maintained into the 1980s. However, Ontario data[41] show that deflated inputs per patient-day and per admission have been rising faster since 1981 as compared to the period between 1967 and 1981. Inputs have been driven up in part because wages have risen faster in the hospital sector than in the general economy. Recently in Ontario, there have been double-digit wage increases for registered nurses, which could accelerate the increase in real inputs per patient-day. Skill mix is also a factor: for any given admission, more highly skilled personnel (or inputs) are applied. Lastly, there is increasing use of day surgery and other ambulatory care alternatives, which appears—paradoxically—to be accelerating the cost spiral by clearing low-intensity bed-days and allowing more high-intensity throughput.

The Canadian system accordingly faces the challenge of reducing the average per capita number of hospital bed-days—a goal already achieved in America.[42] Both systems must contain growth in inputs or service intensity per patient-day—a particular problem in the American hospital sector. As shown in Table 2.3, physician costs as a percentage of GNP are also lower in Canada. The population–physician ratio is only slightly higher in Canada,[43] hence the difference stems largely from lower average gross incomes. A recent analysis confirms that the lower gross incomes partly reflect lower fees, with higher numbers of services per practitioner as would be expected given the higher per capita claim rate.[44] Indeed, in the last 20 years American fees have increased about 20% in real dollar terms, while Ontario fees have decreased by the same amount. This is clearly attributable to the single-payer or monopsony position of provincial governments, and the introduction of collective bargaining over medical payments.

Average *gross* earnings are strikingly discrepant for physicians in Canada and the USA, with six-figure differences commonplace in many specialties. Average *net* income differences are smaller, amounting to about US $50 000 per year on a national basis.[43] The narrowing of the net income differential is due to higher overheads in America, notably administrative expenses and much higher malpractice insurance premiums. Net incomes are similar in most non-procedural specialties, but major gaps emerge for procedure-intensive medical disciplines (e.g. cardiology or gastroenterology) and surgical specialties. These differences are attributable to much higher procedural fees in America.[43,44]

Of interest, between 1971 and 1989 there was a sevenfold increase in malpractice claims filed against Canadian physicians, and malpractice insurance premiums have quadrupled in the last several years. Nonetheless, the number of incidents per physician is five times higher in the USA, and the average malpractice insurance premium nine times higher.[45]

Within a broader societal context, net incomes of full-time private practitioners in Canada have averaged around four to five times the national average of wages and salaries for the past 50 years.[7] Current figures remain in the low end of this range, slightly higher than just prior to the first provincial Medicare plan (1962) when the net taxable medical income was about 3.8 times the national average of wages and salaries.

MEDICAL MANPOWER

Medical manpower growth in both Canada and the USA has vastly outstripped population growth.[43,46,47] From 1961 to 1986 the growth in supply of physicians exceeded population growth in Canada by 2.3% per year, compounding to create a striking increase in active physician manpower that is ongoing. Doctor–population ratios in Canada and the USA are now both well under 500 : 1. Each country has persisting problems with inadequate planning leading to under- and over-supply of various categories of practitioners, combined with endemic geographic maldistribution that has only been partly ameliorated by the major expansion in physician numbers. Incentive programmes are widely used to draw practitioners to rural areas, with variable results. The province of Quebec has combined carrot and stick, paying inflated, standard, or reduced fees to new practitioners, depending on the physician density in the locale where they choose to open an office. Legislation introduced in 1991 gives the Quebec government even more sweeping powers to direct physicians in place of practice, and is being protested vigorously by organised medicine. Another province, British Columbia, attempted to refuse all billing privileges to new practitioners entering areas deemed overserviced, but the legislation was struck down by the courts with reference to the Canadian Charter of Rights and Freedoms. Some legal and policy analysts believe that redrafted legislation would withstand the test of another court challenge, and further attempts at regional quotas on the numbers of practitioners allowed to bill a given provincial Medicare plan appear likely in future. In both nations, an underlying problem is failure to define manpower targets, i.e. to decide what exactly constitutes a manpower shortfall or excess.

In Canada, as in America, paediatrics and some surgical specialties (notably obstetrics/gynaecology) have made inroads into primary care. However, Canadian primary care is still delivered predominantly by GPs or family doctors, unlike America, where general internists deliver much adult primary care—one source of savings in the Canadian system. Paramedical personnel in diverse categories, however, are used suboptimally in Canada. This is due to limitations on payment provisions for delegated acts under the provincial plans, as well as a lack of planning directed at cutting medical manpower growth in favour of paramedical alternatives. In the presence of ample physician supply, governments understandably fear that nurse-practitioners would become an add-on expense, rather than a source of cost savings.

Governments have emphasised the role of a rising doctor–population ratio in generating increased service utilisation per capita, implicitly or explicitly invoking the theory of supplier-induced demand.[48] In provinces with a high doctor–population ratio, such as Ontario and British Columbia, organised medicine has also come to accept the drawbacks of unchecked manpower growth, if only because of the inevitable pressure that results on average incomes. However, until recently there has been a lack of willingness to address the root problem and reduce medical school enrolments. Such reductions are politically unpalatable, in part because residents of remote areas continue to suffer from 'starvation in the midst of plenty' due to maldistribution. A related problem is that even should one province reduce its output of new physicians, interprovincial migration of practitioners cannot be proscribed under the Charter of Rights and Freedoms. Hence, any move to reduce medical school output either needs to be national in scope, or coupled with billing number restrictions to discourage in-migration of practitioners from other provinces. The fiscal crisis of 1992, together with an influential manpower policy analysis by two leading health economists,[49,50] has finally catalysed a national consensus among health ministers to proceed with a reduction in medical school enrolment and postgraduate training positions. These reductions are being implemented in 1993, and an informal national strategy on other policies (e.g. billing restrictions) is also starting to emerge.

MANAGEMENT METHODS AND ALTERNATIVE DELIVERY INITIATIVES

Albeit perhaps not dissimilar to the 'usual, customary, and reasonable' fees of American insurers, the standardised fee schedules and bans on extra charges in Canada do curtail medical economic autonomy. Nonetheless, Canadian practitioners have largely escaped the managerial revolution working its way through the American system.[7,31,51] Government action may be precipitated by the rising per capita utilisation of medical services. For example, between fiscal 1978–79 and 1987–88, the number of claims per capita in Ontario rose from 6.3 to 9.3. In British Columbia, age-specific increases in the per capita use of medical services between 1974–75 and 1985-86 were 3% per annum, with a doubling in the use of specialist services by the elderly during the decade in question.[52] This phenomenon has contributed to the maintenance of medical incomes despite the constraints on fees and major growth in physician numbers. Quebec has accordingly capped payments to physicians on a quarterly basis for several years as a means of containing utilisation-related cost increases. Latterly, other provinces have implemented billing caps and utilisation controls; in the latter, fees can be pro-rated or the next fiscal year's negotiated fee increase rolled back in lockstep with rises in utilisation of medical services. For example, the 1991 agreement between the Ontario Medical Association (OMA) and provincial government entrenched both fixed billing caps (billings from $400 000 to $450 000 a year are reduced by one-third, and those beyond $450 000 by two-thirds), and reductions in fees if demographic-adjusted utilisation growth goes beyond a predetermined threshold.

While these measures constitute overall curbs on income growth due to utilisation increases, the direct management and review of clinical services is minimal. Practitioners in the Canadian fee-for-service sector face review of service claims based primarily on statistical outliers in billing patterns and occasional random sampling of patients. There are a few exceptions, such as the utilisation management mechanisms applied by the Greater Victoria Hospital Society in British Columbia. The latter entails review with explicit criteria based on the Medical Illness Severity Grouping System or Medisgroups[25]—a system popular in American institutions. However, as a general rule, one finds no routine use of case management systems, no pre-service or pre-admission authorisations, no mandatory second-opinion programmes, no monitoring of outcomes data by prepayment agencies, and no prepayment bodies such as health maintenance organisations (HMOs) with contractual arrangements and shared financial risk for providers.[7,25]

The Canadian Medicare system has actually curbed managerial intervention in various unintended ways. With billing privileges apparently upheld by law, and first dollar coverage universally available in an open-ended fee-for-service system, there its little incentive for physicians to accept salaried arrangements[7,25]—a contrast with the current American situation.[53] Similarly, there is no reason for consumers to accept the restrictions on choice of practitioner and hospital that are inherent in American HMOs.[25] Indeed, the 1984 federal legislation that penalised user charges incidentally precluded bearing of financial risk by subscribers; financial 'lock-in' as practised by most American HMOs is therefore impossible. Any attempt by government to change these ground rules of prepayment could precipitate major political conflicts with providers and consumers alike. Furthermore, in Canada, private prepayment organisations cannot purchase public hospitals or attempt any of the vertical and horizontal integrative strategies used in America by corporate conglomerates and large HMO chains alike.

The Ontario provincial government is now encouraging experimentation with capitated prepayment arrangements that will be extended to hospital and specialty services. These Canadianised HMOs are called 'comprehensive health organisations'.[25] However, unless there are legislative changes, such bodies will inevitably be even less restrictive than the so-called 'open-ended' HMOs in the USA which are rapidly emerging as a popular alternative to traditional HMOs, with their stringent lock-in provisions and restricted choice of providers.

Within hospitals, the global budgetary system has contributed to the under-management of clinical services. The overhead savings from global budgets are undeniable, but lump sum prospective payments preclude the necessity for careful per case and per diem tracking of costs. A balanced budget at year end is the hallmark of success, independent of how many patients were efficiently and effectively served. Throughput funding bonuses are available, but have only a minor impact. More recently, Ontario has moved to a system called 'resource intensity weights', wherein case-mix adjustment is made to the lump sum payments. This system is less administratively cumbersome than the diagnosis-related group approach to hospital prospective payment in America's public insurance plans. However, it also lacks the direct per case management incentives, its impact on funding is small, and resultant changes in organisational behaviour remain uncertain. Lack of incentives aside, financial pressures alone have catalysed major shifts in the hospital sector as outlined above.

On the broader front of technolgy and practice patterns assessment, Canada has again moved slowly.[54] During the late 1980s several provinces had technology assessment bodies, but budgets were typically less than half a million dollars a year, and only a handful of drugs, devices and programmes were reviewed annually. Perhaps the most successful government-sponsored experiment is the Canadian Task Force on the Periodic Health Examination;[55] it has generated guidelines on preventive primary care services for over a decade, and has had an international influence. However, the Canadian Task Force has done little to ensure that its guidelines are implemented. Specialty societies and medical associations have actually taken the greatest initiative in developing guidelines for medical practice and appraising new technologies, usually without financial assistance from government.[54,56] As to practice patterns and outcomes, most provincial Medicare plans have not taken advantage of their enormous databases. They have oriented themselves to paying provider claims, rather than generating information that might help in planning and appraising health care. Manitoba has been the major exception,[57] and other provinces are now belatedly following suit. New developments include multi-million dollar commitments to utilisation research institutes in Saskatchewan and Ontario.

RATIONING HEALTH CARE: CANADA VERSUS AMERICA

Health care rationing can be defined as limitation on the availability of beneficial interventions such that some persons are denied useful services. Price-based self-rationing occurs when persons are deterred from appropriate use of services by inadequate insurance coverage or by direct charges (e.g. co-insurance, deductibles and other user fees). Non-price mechanisms include geography, information or influence, and random variations in quality and availability of services.[58–60] The Oregon approach is a peculiar amalgam of both forms of rationing. What garners academic kudos and media attention is the concept of public involvement in ranking services and withholding benefits for those services that are deemed cost-ineffective or of limited marginal yield.[61] What is often overlooked is the fact that these restrictions do not apply to those who are given more comprehensive coverage through conventional private plans. As such the Oregon plan merely adds a gloss of legitimacy to the fundamental inequity that characterises the modern American health care system.

Waiting lists, often seen as a form of rationing, must actually be appraised individually as to the relative elements of delay versus denial.[40] In fact, no waiting presupposes excess capacity, so that patients of any level of urgency can be treated virtually at once. Whatever the verisimilitude of the theory of supplier-induced demand,[48] it is hard to imagine that practitioner thresholds for hospitalisation and surgery are not affected by unused capacity, particularly when services are delivered in a for-profit hospital. Hence, some queueing may actually be seen as an efficiency-enhancing strategy of delay rather than denial.[40] On the other hand, in the UK, with about 1 million persons awaiting various inpatient services for periods of up to 2 years,[62] queues appear to be part of a policy of implicit denial, cloaked in the ersatz egalitarianism of equal access and universal coverage through the National Health Service. How, then, do Canada and the USA stack up?

Price-rationing occurs implicitly in American health care,

given the millions of persons who lack appropriate coverage. More explicit price-rationing mechanisms are also evident, such as co-insurance or user charges of various kinds. Perhaps the most extreme form of price-based rationing occurs with 'dumping'—the phenomenon whereby American private hospitals turn away uninsured patients.[29,30] Recently attention has also been called to a form of queueing in America: poor and uninsured patients in the emergency departments of public hospitals wait so long that some, despite manifest need, give up and leave.[63,64]

Canada's system, in contrast, embodied a policy thrust to eliminate price or payment as a barrier to receiving basic services. However, implicit *non*-price-rationing has now emerged. Long queues exist for a variety of services: e.g. waits of up to 18 months for hip replacement surgery and 12 months for cataract surgery in some Ontario centres, and delays of 3–6 months for elective coronary bypass surgery in several other provinces.

Perhaps because of the emotional connotations of heart surgery, delays in that realm have caused unfavourable publicity in America for the Canadian system, including a story in the *Wall Street Journal* with the suggestive headline: 'Canadians cross border to save their lives'.[65] The latter referred to the movement of Ontarians to adjacent American centres to avoid delays in open-heart surgery—an unforeseen application of the portability provisions in Canadian health insurance coverage! Responding to the long waiting times, Ontario doctors adopted a scoring system to help assess the priority of patients requiring coronary revascularisation.[66] In British Columbia the situation became so acute that the government itself arranged to send 200 patients to Seattle to reduce the backlog. A new cardiac surgery unit has since opened in British Columbia, while in Ontario, as noted above, a recent 10% expansion in open-heart surgery capacity has largely eliminated delays.[40]

The Canadian experience mirrors other nations where elements of allocation by queue tend to supervene sometime after universal health care with full prepayment is instituted.[60] Funds are constrained relative to unchecked demand, and doctors are left to allocate limited services on a decentralised basis. This latter form of allocating scarce services does have advantages. Provider autonomy is maintained to a greater extent[58,67] than would be the case with more bureaucratised controls, and the exercise of clinical judgement allows priorities to be assigned on the basis of patient need—at least in theory. In actual practice, there is little evidence indicating how queues function, but two studies are pertinent. Morris *et al.* reviewed charts of patients on waiting lists for coronary angiography in Winnipeg, Manitoba, during 1981–82.[68] Not only were adverse events rare, but also patients on the elective waiting list differed strikingly from those who underwent more urgent catheterisation—indicative of practitioners' attempts to put those at higher risk to the head of the queue. More recently, our group reviewed charts of over 400 consecutive patients who underwent coronary angiography in various Toronto centres in 1987–88 when delays in surgery were at their worst.[69] Waiting times and clinical features of patients proceeding to surgery were measured against the consensus criteria for patient ranking noted above.[66] There was consistent evidence across all centres that patients perceived to be at highest risk were streamed to the head of the queue, even though formal triage criteria had yet to be adopted. On the other hand, few clinicians relish this role as informal rationing agents, and fewer still can maintain a perspective that enables them to set aside personal priorities and promote a planning process that makes optimum use of limited resources.[40,58]

In sum, queueing for some specialised services appears to be a reasonably equitable and efficient allocation method, provided that the queues are tightly managed and monitored. Furthermore, in contrast to delayed access to any services among America's uninsured and underinsured,[70] delays in Canada tend to occur only for some specialised services and only after patients have been appraised by a family physician and one or more specialists. Queues can accordingly be governed by two principles: first come, first served; and worst case, first case. Neither principle is likely to be upheld in the current American system.

CHANGING POSITION OF ORGANISED MEDICINE

Organised medicine in Canada appears to be moving towards an acceptance of greater activism in professional self-regulation as the price for maintaining clinical freedom.[71,72] Collegial controls—through setting guidelines or practice standards, innovations in quality assurance, and programmes of physician-controlled utilisation management—are being championed by leaders of both voluntary medical associations and the statutory licensing and discipline agencies.[54,56,71,72] A recurrent theme is that such collegial controls may impinge somewhat on the autonomy of individual providers, but will protect the profession collectively against the longer-term threat of direct managerial interference by government.[72] In this sense, there are parallels between the view of government taken by Canadian physicians, and the view of for-profit insurers, HMOs and corporate health care conglomerates taken by some American commentators.[51]

Tension has arisen at times between the provincial voluntary associations and the statutory licensing and discipline bodies as to how the thrust for better clinical management is to be implemented.[56,72] Peer review processes, with clinical assessors, have been instituted by some of the licensing bodies, but only a small minority of practitioners in any province are ever audited. Furthermore, the mandate of the statutory bodies is largely to deal with the 'bad apples'—almost the antithesis of current thinking on continuous quality improvement in health care. Provincial voluntary associations have rank-and-file support and may thereby be better positioned to promote wide-ranging quality management initiatives, but they lack the authority to implement these initiatives except on a purely voluntary basis. Not surprisingly, one survey of Ontario doctors showed strong preference for clinical guidelines to be developed by the provincial medical association, rather than the statutory licensing body, and there was even less support for direct government involvement in the development and dissemination of clinical guidelines.[73]

The future management role of organised medicine—and by extension, the autonomy of the individual practitioner—remains uncertain. Until recently, governments have sent mixed signals. Even as many senior bureaucrats and ministers across Canada have criticised the profession for its role in misallocation of health care resources, there has been a failure to create educational programmes and management structures that would help clinicians and organised medicine play a more responsible role. One very recent experiment at the provincial level has been the development of a joint management committee in Ontario that brings the medical association and government together on a monthly basis. This committee is linked to a health services research institute, in hopes of providing an evidence-based approach to medical care policy. It is too early to assess the merits of this innovation.

The last several years have also seen much lip service paid in Canada to the importance of consumers in medical decision-making, be it as patients in a clinical context, or as citizens on district health councils and other management bodies. However, only a few delivery structures, such as community health centres, engage physicians as employees directly accountable to boards with strong lay representation. In sum, jockeying for influence continues among medicine, other health care professions, consumer advocates and agencies, hospital administrators and health ministries.

The latter is similar to America, but with some glaring differences. Canada has effectively eliminated the private insurance industry as a force shaping the system, and for-profit corporations do not control general hospitals or medical practices. Whereas individuals in Canada can only express their dissatisfaction at the ballot box, American consumers do have some latitude in choosing their prepayment arrangements. The latter element of choice, however, is limited in America by another major force that has little influence on the Canadian system—employers. Employers, in conjunction with various insurers, have helped drive the current American trend towards increasing management of clinical care. Lastly, whereas clear divisions exist within American organised medicine about the need for, and directions of, health care reform, the Canadian profession has now grappled with the reality of NHI and emerged with a recognition of the need to forge strong organisations as a counterweight to government monopsony power.

SATISFACTION, EQUITY AND OUTCOMES

Waiting lists notwithstanding, surveys of users show that the majority of Canadian citizens are content with the current system.[1,2] The popularity of the Canadian system probably stems from the combination of first dollar coverage, free choice of provider, and personalised attention inherent in the maintenance of a private practice framework for medical care. Satisfaction ratings in Canada were far ahead of the USA in a 1989 survey of three nations, where the majority of American respondents—61%—favoured adopting the Canadian system.[1] A 1990 report found Canadians to be more satisfied with their system than residents of nine other advanced industrial nations; the USA had the lowest ratings despite highest per capita expenditures.[2] At least three other major American surveys replicated these findings in the same year.[74] As to directions for reform, in January 1991 a poll commissioned by the AMA found that 58% favoured extending federal coverage to the uninsured—a plan similar to that proposed by the AMA, while only 31% supported a Canadian-style plan and 11% were unsure.[75] However, these latter results contradict other polls showing that a majority of Americans favour NHI, and appear explicable by framing effects, i.e. respondents were given two choices: a government plan for all that would require a substantial increase in taxes, versus a plan for those currently uninsured that would lead to smaller increase in taxes. No indication of offsetting decreases in costs of private health insurance premiums was offered.

Provider satisfaction with Canadian health insurance should theoretically be high. The system has eliminated bad debts, discomfiting money dealings with patients, and a great deal of paperwork. It has yielded moderately high net incomes for practitioners, maintained a private fee-for-service framework for medical care, and introduced little in the way of direct management challenges to clinical freedom. Providers have nonetheless been demoralised by recurrent fee disputes, the politicisation of health system management, limits on capital renewal for hospitals, slow diffusion of new technologies, lengthening waiting lists for some services, and repeated government claims that medical abuse of the prepayment system is the root cause of runaway costs. Not surprisingly, then, doctors are ambivalent about Canadian Medicare. In a 1986 national survey[35] on attitudes to government health insurance, half of respondents perceived a loss of clinical autonomy, yet 60–65% also had clearly positive perceptions, i.e. basic satisfaction with practice, quality of care in their province the same or better over the preceding decade, and positive effects on patients' health status through improved access due to Medicare. Another national survey performed in 1992 drew only a 28.2% response rate, but results were similar. Over 80% of respondents said the Canadian health care system was excellent or good; only 1% characterised it as poor. Satisfaction with provincial medicare arrangements and income levels was registered by about 60–70% of physicians. While 45% believed the quality of care had deteriorated a lot or a little in recent years, 36% perceived an improvement.[76]

On a societal basis, the goal of equity in health care is better upheld by the Canadian approach—at least superficially. Patients' incomes have been more or less eliminated as an obvious factor in the provision of medical and hospital services, and some studies suggest that universal first-dollar coverage has eliminated class differences in service utilisation. However, a recent review[77] shows that the findings have been inconsistent, and rising consumption of services with rising income is still reported by some studies. Major class differences in mortality and morbidity indices persist in Canada. For example, in 1971 the difference in life expectancy at birth between highest and lowest income quintiles was 6.3 years for men and 2.8 years for women; in 1986 the differences were only slightly smaller, at 5.6 years for men and 1.9 years for women. Differences are even greater when expressed as *disability-free* life expectancy between highest and lowest socioeconomic quintiles. The persistence of class-based differences in health status within Canada—a finding similar to that of Britain's famous Black Report[78]—merely underscores the fact that elimination of obvious financial barriers to health services is not, in itself, enough to guarantee equal health status across classes.

In comparison to America, Canadian indices of population health status such as life expectancy and infant mortality are generally superior. Life expectancy in 1987 was 1.7 and 1.6 years greater in Canada for males and females, respectively, and infant mortality rates are 25% lower in Canada than in the USA at 7.3 per 1000 live births, versus 10.1 per 1000 in 1987.[79] Note, however, that national aggregate data can be misleading. For example, in Los Angeles the 1989 infant mortality rate for blacks was 20.8 per 1000 live births, compared to 7.4 per 1000 for whites—with the latter figure obviously similar to the Canadian average. These data can be looked at in two ways. On the one hand, they emphasise that NHI may be even more important in a society such as America with a larger underclass and more limited social welfare system than Canada. Conversely, there is little evidence that fully insured American middle-class persons have inferior health status indices to Canadians in a similar socio-economic stratum. Indeed, since health care is a relatively minor determinant of aggregate population health indices, such indicators may not be a good reflection of comparative health systems performance.

Better indicators of health system performance might be indices of process and outcome of care for specific conditions. One surgical outcomes study using administrative data sets for various procedures suggested little or no advantages in postoperative mortality for New England compared to the province of Manitoba.[80] A further analysis with longer-term follow-up was more compelling: after case-mix adjustment, long-term survival for nine of ten procedures favoured Manitoba.[81] However, such comparisons are suggestive, but fraught with confounders, and many more Canadian–American studies of the processes and outcomes of medical services are needed. Discrepancies in overall surgical rates as documented in Table 2.4 leave wide open the question: which rate is right?[82] In fact, Canada, like America, shows major small area variations in rates of many surgical procedures.[83] For example, at the level of counties and mid to large-sized municipalities, coronary surgery rates in Ontario during 1989–90 varied sixfold between the highest and lowest areas even after age and sex adjustment. In both countries the question of practice variations remains one of ongoing concern and research, and it appears that NHI has done nothing to create greater homogeneity in practice styles.

THE CHANGING FACE OF FISCAL FEDERALISM

A dominant force in Canadian public life is governmental debt—amounting to over $30 billion in the last federal budget alone, with various provinces running additional debt in the recent recession. Charges for servicing the federal debt are now the second largest federal expenditure, at over $60 billion per year, well ahead of national health expenditures, which sit in third place at almost $38 billion. The federal deficit is being attacked in a number of ways, not least by shifting costs for social and educational programmes to the provinces. These shifts are best understood in the light of past cost-sharing arrangements.

At the inception of Medicare, the amount the federal government paid was directly linked to the cost of the provincial plans. Differing formulae were applied for hospital and medical services, but in both cases the transfer payment was effectively 50% of the population-scaled national average per capita cost of the relevant services. In 1977, a new arrangement was instituted. Cash transfers were cut, and future increases oriented to changes in the GNP rather than the national increase in publicly insured health service expenditures. However, to offset this drop in direct cash transfers, the federal government reduced its personal and corporate income tax rates, allowing provincial governments to levy a larger share on an individualised basis. Equalisation payments were also instituted because the richer provinces gained more from the tax point transfer.[84] These equalisation payments proved inadequate, and in 1982 a further adjustment was made to offset the unequal taxation base of provinces with widely differing per capita incomes.

Starting in 1986 the federal government initiated further decreases in the cash transfers. In fact, in the decade from 1980 to 1990, the average percentage of provincial health expenditures provided by Ottawa dropped from about 45% to 37% and continues to fall. Estimates by the Canadian Hospital Association suggest that between 1986–87 and 1989–90, the cumulative decrease in payments for health services by the federal government was $2.6 billion. A particular concern at present is that poorer provinces will be harder hit by the decrease in federal transfers, and regional disparities will be systematically widened.

The reduction in cash transfers—and plans for their eventual elimination—weakens the ability of the federal government to enforce uniform terms and conditions across Canada. The Canada Health Act, as noted above, provides for dollar-for-dollar penalties in cash transfers to provinces that allow user charges by doctors and hospitals. Although the decision partly signalled its commitment to greater provincial sovereignty, Quebec in 1991 announced that it would defy the Canada Health Act and initiate a $5.00 user fee for patients presenting to hospital emergency rooms who are deemed not to have a problem requiring urgent attention.[85] The federal government was cautious in its responses for fear of exacerbating constitutional tensions, and the Quebec government quietly dropped the proposal. It remains to be seen if other provinces will move to institute user charges as financial pressures mount.

THE FUTURE: CHALLENGES FOR BOTH SYSTEMS

The basic principles of Canadian Medicare are admirable. However, one cannot escape the conclusion that Canada, like America, faces severe challenges in delivering affordable, equitable and effective health care over the coming decade (see Table 2.5). In both nations, cost escalation has consistently outstripped the consumer price index, and internationally Canada is second only to America in per capita health expenditures. System-wide management initiatives by the provincial health ministries have been few. Micro-level utilisation management and quality-assurance mechanisms are underdeveloped. Technology assessment is still in its infancy, and 'small ticket' innovations diffuse into the Canadian system without careful scrutiny. The apparent abolition of price-rationing aside, health status (and perhaps even service utilisation) remains unequal across socio-economic classes. Moreover, although consumers are highly satisfied, excessive waiting lists have emerged for many types of specialised services.

For two decades, Canada has struck a successful but precarious balance between the American and British models of health care delivery. To maintain that balance, the next decade

Table 2.5 Canada versus America: health systems comparison

	USA	Canada
1. Cost control	+	++
2. Equity	+	+++
3. Technological innovation	++++	+
4. System management	+	+
5. Micro-management	+++	+
5. User satisfaction	++	++++
6. Provider satisfaction	++	++

Note: The scale is obviously an arbitrary construct. A rating of '+' is poor performance, while '++++' is top-ranked international performance.

will almost certainly require a major shift in directions (see Table 2.6). Organised medicine is attempting to maintain the profession's leadership role as the necessary changes occur, but individual practitioners seem frustrated with the system and uncertain about the future. Cross-border traffic in health care concepts now looks likely to be in two directions. Even as Americans consider importing the Canadian commitment to universality and comprehensive coverage, Canadian policy-makers have begun importation of American management strategies. Dialogue between Canadian and American consumers, providers, policy analysts and policy-makers appears increasingly relevant during this period of rapid evolution in the politics and prepayment of health care.

Table 2.6 Some future directions for health care in both nations

1. Critical appraisal of many accepted but unvalidated practices
2. Analysis of delivery patterns, e.g. to identify and reduce small area variations in service rates, and otherwise enhance the ratio of appropriate to inappropriate care
3. Stringent assessment of new technologies with related clinical guideline development
4. Continued development and dissemination of physician-friendly quality-assurance mechanisms
5. Greater consumer participation in clinical decision-making and provider participation in system-wide management
6. Growth in alternative institutions and delivery systems, e.g. day surgery, home care, birthing centres, hospices, multi-speciality and multi-disciplinary clinics
7. Outreach programmes for the underprivileged to reduce socio-economic inequality in health status
8. Increased experimentation with provider payment mechanisms other than open-ended fee-per-item-of-service
9. More sophisticated prospective funding of hospitals, with fairer case-mix weighting
10. More effective manpower planning, including better use of paramedical personnel and allied health professionals
11. Continued efforts to redress maldistribution of doctors
12. Renewed commitment to public health education and other community health promotion activities

ACKNOWLEDGEMENTS

This chapter is dedicated to the memory of a colleague and friend, Dr Adam Linton, who died in office as the 1991–92 President of the Ontario Medical Association. The author would like to thank his colleagues at the Sunnybrook Clinical Epidemiology Unit and the Institute for Clinical Evaluative Sciences in Ontario for many helpful suggestions, and Dr Art King of Lehigh University's Canadian Studies Program for his hospitality. The author alone, however, is responsible for all sins of omission and commission. An earlier and much shorter version of this article was published in *Current Surgery* (April 1991). The present chapter has also been revised and updated from the article which appeared in *Health Economics* in 1992.

REFERENCES

1. Blendon, R. J. and Taylor, H. Views on health care: public opinion in three nations. *Health Affairs* 1989; **8** (Spring): 149–157.
2. Blendon, R. J., Leitman, R., Morrison, I. and Donelan, K. Satisfaction with health systems in ten nations. *Health Affairs* 1990; **9** (Summer): 185–192.
3. American College of Physicians. Access to health care. *Annals of Internal Medicine* 1990; **112**: 641–661.
4. Sullivan, P. The AMA looks north with fear and loathing. *Canadian Medical Association Journal* 1990; **142**: 50–51.
5. Tuohy, C. Conflict and accommodation in the Canadian health care system. In: R. G. Evans and G. L. Stoddart (eds) *Medicare at Maturity: Achievements, Lessons and Challenges*, Calgary, University of Calgary Press, 1986, 393–434.
6. Horowitz, G. *Canadian Labour in Politics*, Toronto, University of Toronto Press, 1968 (passim).
7. Naylor, C. D. *Private Practice, Public Payment: Canadian Medicine and the Politics of Health Insurance, 1911–1966*, Montreal, McGill–Queen's University Press, 1986.
8. Roper, W. L. Financing health care: a view from the White House. *Health Affairs* 1989; **8** (Winter): 97–102.
9. Dukakis, M. S. The states and health care. *New England Journal of Medicine* 1992; **327**: 1090–1092.

10. Miles, S. H., Lurie, N. and Quam Caplan, A. Health care reform in Minnesota. *New England Journal of Medicine* 1992; **327**: 1092–1094.
11. Taylor, M. G. *Health Insurance and Canadian Public Policy. The Seven Decisions that Created the Canadian Health Insurance System*, Montreal, McGill–Queen's University Press, 1979.
12. Shillington, C. H. *The Road to Medicare in Canada*, Toronto, Del Graphics, 1972.
13. Taylor, M. G. The organization and administration of the Saskatchewan hospital services plan. PhD thesis, University of California at Berkeley, 1948.
14. Naylor, C. D. Canada's first doctors' strike: medical relief in Winnipeg, 1932–4. *Canadian Historical Review* 1986; **LXVII (2)**: 151–180.
15. Badgley, R. F. and Wolfe, S. *Doctors' Strike: Medical Care and Conflict in Saskatchewan*, Toronto, Macmillan, 1967.
16. Gruending, D. *Emmett Hall: Establishment Radical*, Toronto, Macmillan, 1985, 14, 17, 52–67, 70, 78–83.
17. National Council of Welfare. *Medicare: The Public Good and Private Practice*, Ottawa, Supply and Services, 1982.
18. Hall, E. M. *Canada's National-Provincial Health Program for the 1980s: A Commitment for Renewal*, Ottawa, Supply and Services, 1980.
19. Heiber, S. and Deber, R. Banning extra-billing in Canada: just what the doctor didn't order. *Canadian Public Policy* 1987; **13**: 62–74.
20. Tuohy, C. Medicine and the state in Canada: the extra-billing issues in perspective. *Canadian Journal of Political Science* 1988; **21(2)**: 267–296.
21. Kane, R. A. and Kane, R. L. The feasibility of universal long-term care benefits: ideas from Canada. *New England Journal of Medicine* 1985; **312**: 1357–1364.
22. Maxwell, R. J. Financing health care: lessons from abroad. *British Medical Journal* 1988; **296**: 1423–1426.
23. Morgan, P. P. and Cohen, L. Community health centres: do they pose a threat to fee-for-service medicine? *Canadian Medical Association Journal* 1991; **144**: 765–768.
24. Hastings, J. E. F. Organized ambulatory care in Canada: health service organizations and community health centers. *Journal of Public Health Policy* 1986; **6(3)**: 239–247.
25. Lamb, M., Deber, R., Naylor, C. D. and Hastings, J. E. F. *Managed Care in Canada: The Toronto Hospital's Proposed Comprehensive Health Organization*, Ottawa, Canadian Hospital Association Press, 1991.

26. Battista, R. N. and Spitzer, W. O. Adult cancer prevention in primary care: contrasts among primary care practice settings in Quebec. *American Journal of Public Health* 1983; **73**: 1040–1041.
27. Abelson, J. and Lomas, J. Do health service organisations and community health centres have higher disease prevention and health promotion levels than fee-for-service practices? *Canadian Medical Association Journal* 1990; **142**: 575–581.
28. Ginzberg, E. Health care reform: where are we and where should we be going? *New England Journal of Medicine* 1992; **327**: 1310–1312.
29. Schiff, R. L., Ansell, D. A., Schlosser, J. E., Idris, A. H., Morrison, A. and Whitman, S. Transfers to a public hospital: a prospective study of 467 patients. *New England Journal of Medicine* 1986; **314**: 552–557.
30. Reed, W. G., Cawley, K. A. and Anderson, R. J. The effect of a public hospital's transfer policy on patient care. *New England Journal of Medicine* 1986; **315**: 1428–1432.
31. Evans, R. G., Lomas, J., Barer, M. L. *et al.* Controlling health expenditures: the Canadian reality. *New England Journal of Medicine* 1989; **320**: 571–577.
32. Schieber, G. J. and Poullier, J.-P. International health spending: issues and trends. *Health Affairs* 1991; **10** (Spring): 106–116.
33. Coyte, P. C. Current trends in Canadian health care: myths and misconceptions in health economics. *Journal of Public Health Policy* 1990; **11(2)**: 169–188.
34. *National Health Expenditures in Canada 1975–1985*, Ottawa, Minister of Supply and Services, 1987.
35. Stevenson, H. M., Williams, A. P. and Vayda, E. Medical politics and Canadian Medicare: professional response to the Canada health act. *Milbank Quarterly* 1988; **66(1)**: 65–104.
36. Himmelstein, D. U. and Woolhandler, S. Cost without benefit: administrative waste in US health care. *New England Journal of Medicine* 1986; **314**: 441–445.
37. Woolhandler, S. and Himmelstein, D. U. The deteriorating administrative efficiency of the US health care system. *New England Journal of Medicine* 1991; **324**: 1253–1258.
38. Newhouse, J. P., Anderson, G. and Roos, L. L. Hospital spending in the United States and Canada. *Health Affairs* 1988; **7** (Winter): 7–16.
39. Anderson, G. M., Newhouse, J. P. and Roos, L. L. Hospital care for elderly patients with diseases of the circulatory system: a comparison of hospital use in the United States and Canada. *New England Journal of Medicine* 1989; **321**: 1443–1448.

40. Naylor, C. D. A different view of queues in Ontario. *Health Affairs* 1991; **10** (Fall): 110–128.
41. Detsky, A. S., O'Rourke, K., Naylor, C. D., Stacey, S. R. and Kitchens, H. M. Containing Ontario's hospital costs under universal insurance in the 1980s: what was the record? *Canadian Medical Association Journal* 1990; **142**: 565–572.
42. Schwartz, W. B. and Mendelsohn, D. N. Hospital cost containment in the 1980s: hard lessons learned and prospects for the 1990s. *New England Journal of Medicine* 1991; **324**: 1037–1042.
43. Iglehart, J. K. Canada's health care system faces its problems. *New England Journal of Medicine* 1990; **322**: 562–568.
44. Fuchs, V. R. and Hahn, J. S. How does Canada do it? A comparison of expenditures for physicians' services in the United States and Canada. *New England Journal of Medicine* 1990; **323**: 884–890.
45. Coyte, P. C., Dewees, D. N. and Trebilcock, M. J. Medical malpractice: the Canadian experience. *New England Journal of Medicine* 1991; **324**: 89–93.
46. Iglehart, J. K. Canada's health care system: addressing the problem of physician supply. *New England Journal of Medicine* 1986; **315**: 1623–1628.
47. Lomas, J. and Barer, M. L. And who shall represent the public interest? The legacy of Canadian health manpower policy. In: R. G. Evans and G. L. Stoddart (eds) *Medicare at Maturity: Achievements Lessons and Challenges,* Calgary, University of Calgary Press, 1986, 221–286.
48. Reinhardt, U. The theory of physician-induced demand: reflections after a decade. *Journal of Health Economics* 1985; **4**: 187–193.
49. Barer, M. L. and Stoddart, G. L. Toward integrated medical resource policies for Canada. *Canadian Medical Association Journal* 1992; **146**: 347–351, 697–700, 1169–1174, 1549–1554, 1919–1924.
50. Barer, M. L. and Stoddart, G. L. Toward integrated medical resource policies for Canada. *Canadian Medical Association Journal* 1992; **147**: 33–38, 305–312, 617–623, 999–1005, 1325–1329, 1653–1660.
51. Grumbach K. National health insurance in America: can we practice with it? Can we continue to practice without it? *Western Journal of Medicine* 1989; **151**: 210–216.
52. Barer, B. L., Pulcins, I. R., Evans, R. G., Hertzman, C., Lomas, J. and Anderson, G. M. Trends in use of medical services by the elderly in British Columbia. *Canadian Medical Association Journal* 1989; **141**: 39–45.
53. Korcok, M. US doctors flocking to salaried employment. *Canadian Medical Association Journal* 1987; **136**: 73–75.

54. Linton, A. L. and Naylor, C. D. Organized medicine and technology assessment: lessons from Ontario. *New England Journal of Medicine* 1990; **323**: 1463–1467.
55. Canadian Task Force on the Periodic Health Examination: the periodic health examination. *Canadian Medical Association Journal* 1979; **121**: 1194–1254.
56. Linton, A. L. and Peachey, D. K. Guidelines for medical practice: 1. The reasons why; 2. A possible strategy. *Canadian Medical Association Journal* 1990; **143**: 485–490, 629–632.
57. Manitoba has benefited from the pioneering work of Noralou and Leslie Roos. See, for example, Roos, L. L., Sharp, S. M. and Wajda, A. Assessing data quality: a computerized approach. *Social Science and Medicine* 1989; **28**: 175–182.
58. Naylor, C. D. and Linton, A. L. Allocation of health care resources: a challenge for the medical profession. *Canadian Medical Association Journal* 1986; **134**: 333–340.
59. Aaron, H. and Schwartz, W. B. Rationing health care: the choice before us. *Science* 1990; **247**: 418–422.
60. Schwartz, W. B. and Aaron, H. J. Rationing hospital care: lessons from Britain. *New England Journal of Medicine* 1984; **310**: 52–56.
61. Kaplan, R. M. *The Hippocratic Predicament: Affordability, Access, and Accountability in American Medicine*, San Diego, Academic Press, 1993.
62. Rigge, M. *Guide to Hospital Waiting Lists 1990*, London, College of Health, 1990.
63. Baker, D. W., Stevens, C. D. and Brook, R. H. Patients who leave a public hospital emergency department without being seen by a physician. Causes and consequences. *Journal of the American Medical Association* 1991; **266**: 1085–1090.
64. Bindman, A. B., Grumbach, K., Keane, D., Rauch, L. and Luce, J. M. Consequences of queuing for care at a public hospital emergency department. *Journal of the American Medical Association* 1991; **266**: 1091–1096.
65. Barnes, J. A. Canadians cross border to save their lives. *Wall Street Journal* December 12, 1990.
66. Naylor, C. D., Baigrie, R. S., Goldman, B. S. and Basinski, A. Revascularisation panel, Consensus methods group. Assessment of priority for coronary revascularisation procedures. *Lancet* 1990; **335**: 1070–1073.
67. Mechanic, D. Approaches to controlling the costs of medical care: short-range and long-range alternatives. *New England Journal of Medicine* 1978; **298**: 249–254.
68. Morris, A. L., Roos, L. L., Brazauskas, R. and Bedard, D.

Managing scarce services: a waiting list approach to cardiac catheterization. *Medical Care* 1990; **28**: 784–792.
69. Naylor, C. D., Levinton, C. M., Wheeler, S. and Hunter, L. Queueing for coronary surgery during severe supply–demand mismatch in a Canadian referral centre: a case study of implicit rationing. *Social Science and Medicine* 1993; in press.
70. Weissman, J. S., Stern, R., Fielding, S. L. and Epstein, A. M. Delayed access to health care: risk factors, reasons, and consequences. *Annals of Internal Medicine* 1991; **114**: 325–331.
71. Linton, A. L. and Peachey, D. K. Utilization management: a medical responsibility. *Canadian Medical Association Journal* 1989; **141**: 283–286.
72. Naylor, C. D. and Hollenberg, A. A. Practice guidelines and professional autonomy in a universal health insurance system: the case of tissue plasminogen activator in Ontario. *Social Science and Medicine* 1990; **31**: 1327–1336.
73. Naylor, C. D., Hollenberg, A. A., Ugnat, A. M. and Basinski A. Coronary thrombolysis, clinical guidelines, and public policy: results of an Ontario practitioner survey. *Canadian Medical Association Journal* 1990; **142**: 1069–1076.
74. Ferris, L. E., Williams, J. I., Llewellyn-Thomas, H. A., Naylor, C. D., Cohen, M. M. and Basinski, A. S. H. Public opinions about health care. *Canadian Medical Association Journal* 1992; **147**: 1133–1137.
75. Wolinsky, H. Americans shy away from Canadian-style health care. *Medical Post* 1991; **27** (April 9): 37.
76. *The Medical Post 1992 National Survey of Canadian Doctors*. Supplement to the Medical Post. Toronto, Maclean-Hunter, Fall 1992.
77. Badgley, R. F. and Wolfe, S. Equity and health care. In: C. D. Naylor (ed.) *Canadian Health Care and the State: A Century of Evolution*, Montreal, McGill–Queen's University Press, 1992, 193–237.
78. Townsend, P. and Davidson, N. (eds) *Inequalities in Health: The Black Report*, Harmondsworth, Penguin, 1982.
79. World Health Organization. *1989 World Health Statistics Annual*, Geneva, WHO, 1989.
80. Roos, L. L., Fisher, E. S., Sharp, S. M., Newhouse, J. P., Anderson, G. and Bubolz, T. A. Postsurgical mortality in Manitoba and New England. *Journal of the American Medical Association* 1990; **263**: 2453–2458.
81. Roos, L. L., Fisher, E. S., Brazauskas, R., Sharp, S. M. and Shapiro, E. Health and surgical outcomes in Canada and the United States. *Health Affairs* 1992; **12**: 56–72.

82. Wennberg, J. E. Which rate is right? *New England Journal of Medicine* 1986; **314**: 310–311.
83. Vayda, E., Barnsley, J. M., Mindell, W. R. and Cardillo, B. Five-year study of surgical rates in Ontario counties. *Canadian Medical Association Journal* 1984; **131**: 111–115.
84. Soderstrom, L. *The Canadian Health System*, London, Croom Helm, 1978, 139–140, 162–164.
85. Pole, K. Feds Now Hint Canada Health Act Disposable. *Medical Post* 1991; **27** (May 7): 1, 72.

CHAPTER 3

Fairness and feasibility in national health care systems

Mark V. Pauly
The Wharton School and the Leonard Davis Institute of Health Economics, Philadelphia, Pennsylvania, USA

INTRODUCTION

Medical care is different from other goods and services in many ways. Medical care affects life and death. To be sure, so do some other goods, at some sufficiently low level of consumption: food, housing in cold climates, and household testing for radon gas are all matters of life and death if consumed infrequently enough. Medical services seem special, however, in that their relationship to life expectancy seems (and probably is) much more direct.

Somewhat surprisingly, a large body of economic research on consumer/patient behaviour strongly suggests that this apparently important difference has relatively little distinctive impact on the shape of the demand curve or demand function for this service. People buy more medical services when they are free than when they have to pay for them; demand curves slope downward. Other things (including price paid and state of health) equal, higher-income people spend more on medical services. The amount of medical care demanded depends on

North American Health Care Policy in the 1990s
Edited by A. King, T. Hyclak, S. McMahon and R. Thornton

'tastes', as well as income, price and the state of one's health. The only really peculiar phenomenon on the demand side seems to come from the fact that consumers have to use agents—health professionals—to advise them on what they should buy. This relationship may function in somewhat bizarre ways, but perhaps people's relationships with other agents, for example auto mechanics and appliance repairmen, would turn out to be equally bizarre, if only their share of gross national product (GNP) were high enough to motivate research.

Where the medical care 'life and death' connection matters the most, I believe, is not so much in how we think about our own use of medical services, but in how we feel about others' use. I use the word 'feel' here in the sense of 'feelings', as opposed to what one might label 'objective reasons', because I believe that our concern for this service does go back to fundamental and elemental empathetic and altruistic concerns that humans have for each others' health.

One manifestation of this concern, as it gets translated into policy discussion, is the issue of equity in health care services use. People are not only concerned about health care equity, of course; they are also concerned about equity in the distribution of income or command over resources, and equity in the use of some other goods or services. Probably those who favour more equity in one also favour more equity in the other. However, I am going to take as given the fact that the distribution of income, in the USA and Canada, is not going to be changed, and is not going to be made more equal. Whether you think that current distribution of income ought to be made more equal (as I do), or whether you would call the current distribution equitable enough, we can probably all agree that we should analyse equity in medical care services under the assumption that a revolution in overall income distribution is not going to happen anytime soon. The fundamental question about equity in medical services then is: in a society which accepts fairly substantial inequality in the distribution of income after taxes and transfers, what do we mean by equity in a particular service like medical services, and what policies might be most appropriate?

Why might one be concerned about fairness with respect to medical care use and cost? The literature distinguishes three broad classes of reasons: two (the most important two) relating to use, and one relating to cost.

The most obvious reason for concern is that unequal use may be a proxy for inappropriately low use. What is low or inappropriate cannot be answered solely based on clinical judgement alone; fundamentally, it depends on the value that taxpayers attach to additional use by people in categories that make them chronic below-average users. Exactly what would constitute a minimum acceptable level of benefits is hard to specify, and probably requires better understanding of the effectiveness of medical care. It also requires assuming, probably illogically, that one can identify a level of use below which disaster occurs and above which benefits are trivial; it requires assuming that nature does make a leap. Even for such binary services as appendectomies, there are variations in the strength of indication for surgery. Nevertheless, the concept of equity as associated with minimising harm from underconsumption of medical care surely captures part of the feeling of many.

A second reason for concern is higher-than-average use by some. It should be noted that putting an upper limit on someone's consumption of purchased medical care (as opposed to public medical care), in a world of unequal incomes, does nothing for overall equity; it simply forces the person to spend his income on other things, and things which are of lower value to him. Inequity is simply squeezed from one object of consumption to another. To be sure, inequity in the use of restaurant meals or travel may not be viewed as so bothersome as inequity in the use of physical examinations, *in vitro* fertilisation, or nursing home care.

The third kind of equity consideration arises when financing arrangements affect the distribution of cost across persons, even when coverage, or use conditional on state of health, is the same. To take an example that will be explored in more detail in what follows: if some people have a higher probability than others of getting an illness, the competitive insurance premiums that will be charged to the first group will be higher than those charged to the second. The result need not be a difference in the use of medical care by sick people, but is likely to lead to greater inequality in the amount of income left to spend on other things. This inequality in disposable income may also be regarded as unfair.

THE DEFINITION OF AND DEMAND FOR FAIRNESS

These are the objects of discussions of fairness, but what is fair? Ethics, rather than economics, is needed to answer this question. I do not propose an amateur investigation of ethical theory, so I will follow the strategy of trying to infer the ethical judgements people seem willing to make, rather than posit ones of my own.

Whatever the idealised ethical standard, however, I will take the position that the concrete manifestation of ethical behaviour does (and arguably should) respond to economic forces. In most circumstances, there is a cost to achieving any ethical goal. Given some goal that admits of degrees, the extent to which it will be reached might well depend on this cost.

The most obvious cost associated with attempts to equalise rewards is the probable attenuation of incentives. The philosopher John Rawls in fact made the potential reduction in output associated with greater equity his rationale for advocating the outcome that maximised the well-being of the worst-off person, rather than the situation of perfect equality.[1]

For a specific good like medical care, this cost is unlikely to be high, simply because total medical spending is not so large a part of total income. However, there are two other costs that might be important: one is most obvious; there can be a bureaucratic administrative cost to trying to produce equity in medical care consumption. The other reason is less obvious, but possibly equally important: when people are different, they will not be happy to consume identical amounts of anything.

What I want to suggest here is that perhaps one reason why the USA has not achieved as much equity in the use of or access to medical services is because improvements in equity have higher costs in the USA. We have no precise measures, but the amount of heterogeneity in demand for medical care and medical insurance in the USA appears to be substantial, as expressed in the variety of different health insurance plans, health maintenance organisations (HMOs), and delivery systems we have fostered.[2] Variation in use of services that arises purely from variation in income is perhaps questionable, but even within income classes there appears to be substantial variation in the amount and type of medical care Americans seek. Some people like HMOs, and choose them to save money, while others stick with good old Blue Cross to avoid hassles and preserve their ability to choose.

An important question is the empirical one: under the appearance of diversity, how much variation in tastes and desires is there? Europeans are mystified at our variety of health care financing and delivery arrangements; they wonder why we discomfort ourselves in making difficult choices, rather than turning things over to a kindly and benevolent bureaucrat. Perhaps we have more distrust of bureaucrats and politicians too (and not without reason), but the main point here is that careful documentation of diversity, and its sources, would help us enormously to understand ourselves. Even if we do confirm diversity, that does not mean that we should not seek equity, but it does mean that the equity ought to be of a different sort than what most other countries have chosen thus far.

There is another cost to achieving equity that Uwe Reinhardt has noted.[3] He points out that the high cost of medical services in the USA may help to explain why we choose to transfer less to the poor, why our safety net is more porous than those in other countries. At the conceptual level, things are not completely straightforward. As Thomas Grannemann has noted, when medical costs rise relative to income, those who would not be viewed as poor enough to need help when care is cheap may now be regarded as deserving.[4]

What is perhaps more puzzling is the source of this higher price. To the extent that it represents higher input prices, as I will argue below, then Reinhardt's argument holds. To the extent it represents a higher average quality or intensity of care chosen by non-poor people, and there is some evidence for this as well, there is no direct reason why taxpayers cannot at the same time choose cheaper quality for transfer recipients. Such a two-class approach is something Americans have always denied in rhetoric but practised in reality. Nevertheless, it would be perverse indeed if we chose to avoid providing any assistance to the poor just because we are unwilling to pay the price of high-tech care—but stranger things have happened.

Then if we assume that some do want more than others, or something different from others, a system such as the Canadian one will not satisfy these different desires. Slightly more formally, providing just one quantity or quality of care leaves both those who want more and those who want less unsatisfied. To be sure, making just one version of something can cause its cost to be lower, if only because of a reduction in administrative cost. But in this case, as in many others, cost reduction is only an accounting curiosity; it does not imply that the outcome is better.

WHAT IS EQUITY?

Moving the quantity of some good that is below the appropriate quantity toward that level will generally be regarded as desirable if it is not too costly. But there apparently can be a difference of opinion when we think of the possibility of someone receiving a quantity which is above the minimum acceptable amount. If the person who gets more pays the full cost of what he gets, and if his or her additional purchase does not raise the price that others pay, then prohibiting such purchases provides no benefits to those who use less. It only deprives those who use more of an opportunity to buy something they find more valuable than other ways of spending their money. The President's Commission on Ethics took a straightforward position on this matter.[5] It defined equity as not a ceiling above which no one's consumption can rise, but rather as a floor below which no one's consumption should be allowed to sink. This definition would perhaps not be found acceptable in Canada, where there appears to be much more emphasis on equality of access per se, rather than simply improved access for those who lack it. Indeed, the Canadian system makes it illegal to insure privately to supplement the public payments for publicly insured services.

The USA, in contrast, appears to have accepted a 'bottom-up' view of equity in medical services, since the Capron commission's view has not been challenged. I have to admit some personal disquiet at the thought that I might buy some medical care of small but positive benefit for my family which a Medicaid programme may decide that it cannot afford. But I have even more disquiet at the thought of prohibiting such purchase, of causing unnecessary suffering, just for the sake of an abstract principle. The principle, of course, is equity, but the rationale for it is not only abstract but obscure. It is hard to avoid the conclusion that it is based on envy, and the USA has never cultivated a culture of envy. There is obviously no way to use economics, common sense, or an easy and transparent philosophy to tell you how you should feel on this question. It is, however, important to note its absolutely central role in the debate on fairness, even though that role is often obscured by slogans or sloppy rhetoric.

To be sure, even if one accepts the notion that 'top-down' as well as 'bottom-up' equity is desirable, that need not imply complete levelling. It could be achieved by taxing spending above some limit, and even using the proceeds to pay for care for low users; the principle need not be, and should not be, absolute, since the gain from equalising the last dollar of spending is surely vanishingly small, and the loss from prohibiting use of substantial benefit is great.

Things are more difficult when additional purchases by some push up the price that others must pay; the quintessential example of this case is the situation in which the best doctor in town can be bid away from low income people if we permit private purchases. More generally, this will happen when long-run supply curves slope upward. Straightforward economics would note that, if the doctor really can only serve a limited number of his patients, and if his skills cannot be reproduced at uniform cost, then the ideal arrangement is to provide his services to those for whom they are most valuable, and to compensate the others who were bid out of the market by a direct transfer.

The problem arises when the person who loses does not receive the transfer. In the ordinary operation of a market, payment would stay as part of the provider's income—a rent in excess of the amount needed to render the service rather than not render it at all. If one sports team bids up the salary of a player on another team, the losing team is not usually paid off—only the player. But the problem with superstars must be a minor one in medicine and, in any event, not capable of a fully equitable solution, precisely because the best doctor's skills cannot be evenly spread over all patients in town.

In what follows I am going to take a bottom-up view of equity, and I am going to assume that, in a sufficiently long run, supply curves are horizontal. That is, I will assume that some can buy more without raising the price paid by those who buy less. The reader who is unwilling to make either of these assumptions will not arrive at the same conclusions as I do in what follows.

THE COST OF TAXATION

There is another cost to achieving equity associated with tax-financed national health insurance. Any attempt to increase equity, whether applied to medical services or to wealth in general, has to involve the imposition of compulsory payments on some in order to make transfers to others. And those compulsory payments need to be higher for those with higher wealth. In short, some kind of income or wealth tax is necessary. The fact that funds are raised through taxes—through payments that are unrelated to the benefits received—means that there will be a distortion in incentives. In contrast, for products sold in the market there is no distortion because the buyer sacrifices resources in order to get the good directly.

To economists, these distortions are not just theoretical, they are real. In some cases, the reality can be grasped fairly easily. If a well-to-do investor who is heavily taxed decides to take advantage of one of the inevitable loopholes in the tax code, and divert resources from a more productive but heavily taxed investment to a less productive but less heavily taxed one, total productivity of investment, and therefore GNP, obviously falls. Less obvious in practice but reasonably clear in theory is the notion that taxing income reduces the effort that people will apply to activities whose benefits are represented by money income. The investor will not make the effort to locate the best investment. The consultant will not choose to take the last job, but will take time off instead. The worker will decide to paint his house rather than work overtime, even though the value of what he could produce on the job is greater than the (untaxed) value of 'household production', and the spouse will decide not to take a job at all, but instead stick to housework. The problem with these choices is not that GNP will fall, though it will, but that the overall well-being of people in society will decline, precisely because people devote their effort to less heavily taxed activities as a way to reduce their tax burden. But when we all do that and the tax base erodes, the tax rate has to be put higher to raise a given amount of revenues, and the distortion remains behind as an 'excess burden'.

I do not maintain that people are obsessed with avoiding taxes, or that every person distorts his or her behaviour because of taxation. I do make the conventional economic assumption that there is always some choice on the margin, some decision one would have made one way were there no tax but that is changed if taxation is present. That some distortion is possible cannot be denied, but the real policy question is a quantitative one: how bad is it?

That taxes generally distort behaviour is no reason not to tax: even with the distortion, the objects of public expenditure may be sufficiently valuable that it pays to tax and spend. The crucial point, however, is that tax-financed spending is not free.

I am thinking here not so much of the costs of the Internal Revenue Service, or even of the tax advisor/tax preparation costs we taxpayers retaliate with. In general, however, it appears that the excess burden associated with the conventional income tax/general revenue base is more than negligible.

This discussion makes an important comment on one aspect of the debate on the Canadian system and national health insurance. A number of commentators have pointed out that the administrative burden of the US private health insurance system is far from negligible. The private health insurance system as a whole uses up about 14% of premiums to cover its administrative costs, in contrast to about 3–5% for Medicare and less than 1% for the systems in Canada. Most of the difference seems to be due to selling and premium billing costs, since large private groups in the USA are able to equal the Medicare percentage. The USA average is pulled up by a very high percentage, sometimes as much as 50%, on the small fraction of coverage that is bought on an individual basis.

On the provider side, there are also costs that have to be incurred to itemise the bills for each patient covered by different insurers. In a monopoly system like Canada's, with hospital total budgets subject to approval, there is no need for such detail, and provider administrative costs are lower. Precise estimates are hard to come by here, but some critics of the US system have claimed that US administrative costs under our mixed system exceed what they would have been under a Canadian type system by as much as 20% of premiums. This is not enough to make a massive dent in total cost growth, but it would be enough, if it could be captured, to pay for all of the care currently used by the uninsured.

The logic seems impeccable; administrative 'waste' is such a tangible additional cost of the US system, which a fully public system such as the Canadian one could avoid. The discussion above about excess burden shows, however, that a tax-financed public monopoly is not all pure gain. In particular, if equity dictates that financing of the public system be based on wealth or ability to pay, then it will cost something to shift resources from the private to the public sector. This cost will not show up in accounting ledgers, but it will show up in the total output of the economy. To be sure, not all taxes need impose this burden. A tax which does not depend on wealth—a head tax—would not distort behaviour. But such taxes are usually regarded as wildly inequitable. However, as we shall see in more detail below, some of the ways that have been proposed for financing steps toward improved equity in medical services in the USA are virtually the same as head taxes. For the present, it is sufficient to note that Canada does not use head taxes to finance its national health care.

So if we are to copy the Canadian system in order to obtain the benefit of a lower administrative percentage, we have to pay the cost of a higher excess burden. How high is this cost? There have been, to my knowledge, no estimates of the marginal excess burden cost of the Reagan tax structure, and certainly there have been no estimates for the post-1990 tax increase structure. Estimates have, however, been provided for the early 1980s tax structure. These estimates are, of course, subject to error in estimation, since they require estimating how behaviour would be distorted—how the supply of taxed inputs would change—with a given marginal tax rate, compared to the situation with a lower rate. The estimates assume that the tax base is the one we actually use at the Federal level, relying heavily on individual income and payroll taxes, with modest reliance on the corporation income tax. Estimates of the marginal excess burden have been provided by Shoven and Whalley, and they are in the range of 20%.[6] That is, it is estimated that moving an additional dollar of expenditure from the private to the public sector reduces the value of other output by about 20 cents.

The Reagan era changes in taxes would affect these estimates, but it is not so easy to say how. The cuts in nominal marginal personal income tax rates presumably reduce the excess burden cost, since the cost rises with the marginal tax rate. However, closing loopholes, which the Reagan tax 'cut' also did, is more ambiguous. Loopholes cause distortions, but they may also lower the effective marginal rate if they become more numerous as incomes rise. In addition, the payroll tax for

Social Security and Medicare was raised during this period, as was the maximum wage income subject to tax. On balance, my guess—and it is only a guess—is that the marginal excess burden either stayed the same or fell slightly.

The important point here is that the order of magnitude of the excess burden cost is roughly similar to the order of magnitude of the excess administrative cost; they are both about 20%. More research on this question would definitely help, but my preliminary conclusion is that the higher administrative cost of the current system and the higher excess burden cost of a Canadian-style system appear to wash; there would be neither gains nor losses from the move as far as these considerations are concerned. In this sense, the desire to retain equity in the tax structure, to have the rich pay their 'fair share', as some (who seem to know more than I about what 'fair' is) put it, is a cost to achieving greater equity in the consumption of medical services and greater equity in after-tax income. The key question is whether the movement of some or all of medical spending to the public sector is accompanied by a decision to alter the amount of redistribution undertaken.

One final point. There are some other things we get from the administrative cost of private health insurance which ought also to be mentioned. For one thing, as my colleague Patricia Danzon has noted, some of the administrative cost goes towards cost containment efforts.[7] One would call a cost containment effort successful if the cost of administering the effort were less than the amount of benefit payments saved. Paradoxically, however, such an action would increase administrative costs, reduce benefit payments, and so raise the administrative cost percentage. Such an increase would be meaningless as an indicator of comparative efficiency.

Finally, and perhaps most fundamentally, selling and administrative costs are the price we pay for having choices. Restaurant meals could be a lot cheaper, and both cashier and waiter time saved, if all restaurants served the same thing. Meat loaf may, however, not be to everyone's taste, and the same might be said of a particular style of medical care. The real issue is something already noted above: how much diversity there is in demands for insurance coverage, for the style or type of care, and for the degree of aggression in cost containment, and for the ability to bail out and switch doctors when you get dissatisfied. My own perception is that there is a lot of diversity. I know there is a lot of diversity right now, and I do not think it is all due to disequilibrium or distorted prices (though some may be). The fundamental empirical fact that could help enormously to settle the national health insurance controversy would be a measure of the degree of variation in our citizens' taste for health care and health insurance.

FAIRNESS FEELING SICK

A competitive market must result in each product carrying a price that reflects its true cost. A given health insurance policy held by two persons need not be the same product, even if what is down on paper in black and white is identical. The reason is that the level of anticipated medical expenses may well differ because of variation in health state, in health habits, in family size, in taste for medical care, or in the prevailing level of local medical care prices. Is it unfair for different people to pay different premiums for the same nominal health insurance policy?

The answer to this question, as with so much in economics, is, 'it all depends'. For most people, the critical issue is the reason why expected claims differ. If the reason is bad health habits, or larger family size, or perhaps middle age, many people might be inclined to accept a higher premium as fair. The most problematic of all is variation due to state of health, ideally due to random variation in the state of health that was not caused by the person in that state.

The problem arises because attempts to use markets in medical care to allow people to satisfy their different desires may lead to insurance premiums in which people at higher risk, the likely-to-be-sick, pay more. Insurance will redistribute money from those who do not get sick to those who do, but only if either set have the same probability of getting sick at the beginning. That is, insurance redistributes from the lucky to the unlucky, not from the already-well to the already-sick. However, part of many persons' notion of equity is the thought that those injured by chronic illness should not be further insulted by having to pay insurance premiums fully reflective of the cost of that illness.

Insurers, until recently, claimed that achieving equity was not their problem; more recent statements have suggested that they have assumed responsibility.[8] Insurers achieve a tailoring of premium to risks in two ways. They may actually be able to observe some indicator that is highly correlated with expected claims (including this period's claims). This 'risk rating' is regarded by many as unfair. In addition, certain kinds of low coverage insurance policy may appear to be more attractive to people who know they are low risks but cannot prove it to an insurance company. 'Adverse selection' of low risks into low-coverage policies can lead to premiums closer to risk, though it will distort things by depressing the purchases of low risks, and possibly raising the premiums for generous coverage so much as to drive it out of existence. (Given the health-cost-increasing potential of generous conventional coverage for the middle class, few analysts will shed a tear over its demise.) But the resulting distribution of disposable income, with the chronically ill at a given gross income having less disposable income, might well be regarded as unfair.

At one level, it is unfair in much the same way as any other random reduction in wealth might be regarded as unfair, such as a loss due to a natural calamity or theft, or even an unprofitable business. The general principle we seem to apply to such losses is to encourage their coverage by private insurance and, if the insurance is not present, provide public transfers to offset those losses, but only when they mount high enough to do serious damage to a family's standard of living. Not all random losses are necessarily a matter of social concern requiring full coverage.

When these losses are associated with health insurance premiums, there seems to be a much different standard. Many policy commentators find it desirable (though they may differ on feasibility or practicality) that all should pay the same premium for a given amount of nominal coverage, even though some stand to gain much more from that coverage than others. Until recently, for instance, federally approved HMOs were required to charge the same premium to all, i.e. to community rate. Blue Cross plans historically did the same thing, and the demise of community rating under competitive pressure is usually regarded as a shame. Why the difference in perception?

One answer to this question is that those who face higher premiums may be more likely to decline insurance coverage. The problem with this argument is that it need not be true. For one thing, persons at higher than average risk who know their risk level will buy insurance coverage if faced with a premium that depends on their risk. To be sure, if one charged a premium less than the risk, they would be even more eager to buy, and a premium that exceeds one's income will not be paid. But over a considerable range, the willingness to pay for insurance increases along with the expected loss. A so-called risk-related premium need not discourage persons with above-average risk from purchasing insurance any more than persons of average risk. Moreover, if a higher rate for a bad risk discourages a person from buying insurance, a higher rate for a good risk—a rate higher than the rate that reflects the expected loss—will discourage good risks from buying coverage. To take an extreme (and controversial) example, forcing insurers to sell coverage to people with AIDS at uniform premiums will raise premiums for others, and will discourage some of those others from buying coverage. On theoretical grounds, we cannot say which pricing policy will result in more uninsured. I hasten to add that I am in favour of assistance to persons with AIDS, but I think it should take the form of the explicit transfers I will discuss presently, rather than through community rating.

Another argument is one that has more substance, and that points directly at both appropriate policy and possible market solution. This argument notes that a premium that rises with risk itself forces more risk onto a risk-averse person. To be more concrete: a person who contracts a chronic illness, or even an acute illness with a long span of treatment, faces two risks—the cost of the care immediately received, and the risk of having to pay a higher than average premium for some time in the future. The cost of care immediately received can be covered by insurance, but what of the risk of becoming a high risk?

One need not invoke some notion of equity to get an answer. Instead, one can note that risk-averse people should be willing to buy coverage against this future risk. The relevant question then is simple. What is the appropriate form and amount of insurance against this future loss? Community rating in effect provides full coverage, but is that the right level of coverage?

We can get some insight by considering the tempering of risk rating as a kind of insurance. Why might a person in any circumstances not want to buy full coverage against a loss if that person is risk-averse? One answer is that the insurance might have an administrative cost. Accepting a small risk to avoid paying an insurer to shuffle papers may be a preferred strategy. The other reason is that the insurance may further stimulate the loss-producing behaviour—the so-called 'moral hazard'. This latter reason does not apply to events that are truly random, but it does apply to other events.

It seems implausible at first glance to suppose that community rating should be associated with additional administrative cost. On the contrary, it would seem to be a lot cheaper to use community rating than to go to the effort of figuring out who is at what level of risk, so as to vary premiums. Indeed, the process of assessing and classifying risks, the underwriting function, is itself costly. However, if risk rating is cheap enough that it would pay, and all it requires is that the cost of identifying the good risks be less than the difference in premiums between good risks and other risks, then insurers will naturally seek to avoid selling insurance to persons on whom they expect to lose money. If forced to community rate, they will 'demarket' insurance to higher risks. One can write laws and regulations to prevent this, but enforcing those regulations, and the distorted insurer behaviour that accompanies the regulations, has an administrative cost of its own. Put the person at risk on risk-related premiums, and these costs need not be incurred. Without more information, we cannot tell what is cheaper, but the point remains that, sometimes, people may not suffer from sufficiently modest levels of risk rating.

It is beyond doubt that there are voluntary behaviours that people engage in which may affect the probability that they get ill. Smoking, drinking, not exercising, and other poor health habits can be associated with high claims costs and high premiums. Charging people who engage in such practices a somewhat higher premium seems an eminently sensible way of discouraging bad behaviours. This is not to say that there will not be debate on the degree of volition—alcohol abuse and unsafe sex practices may not be regarded as fully blameworthy. But note that partial insurance coverage only requires that there be some relationship between health habits and insurance premiums, not that the victim be blamed for the full amount of the additional expected loss. In fact, the choice of degree of experience rating could be explicitly keyed to the impact of such rating on behaviour.

Viewed as a matter of rational insurance purchasing by risk-averse persons, some relating of premiums to expected losses seems appropriate. There can be some tapering of relative premiums to account for varying degrees of fault and responsiveness. But community rating seems to reflect abandonment of what could be a useful and cost-effective intervention to encourage health-seeking behaviours.

As with any other kind of health insurance, low-income people might buy too little protection against the risk of becoming a bad risk. The general solution here, however, is not community rating, but rather a programme to ensure that such coverage is in fact purchased. Beyond this, it is not obvious that there is any additional equity dimension, at least not in the long run.

How does one buy insurance coverage against the risk of becoming a bad risk? There are two broad strategies. The one which is probably most common is to purchase insurance as a member of a group which does not drop members at high risk. This strategy requires that the risk be high enough to pool any differential risk. If a group is small, even community rating within the group will be insufficient protection. Choosing an insurance company which may charge a somewhat higher premium but which does not adopt strict underwriting standards for renewal accomplishes the same objective.

The more explicit strategy is to buy an insurance policy with a guaranteed renewability feature. Such features add to the premium charged to ordinary risks, but in return the insurer promises to sell protection at a premium that is the same as it charges standard risks. This follow-on premium cannot rise so much as to drive out those who remain at normal risk. It can involve a somewhat higher premium than what some individual was initially paying. Guaranteed renewability does reduce a person's ability to switch insurers if the person becomes dissatisfied and is at high risk. However, since the great majority of people will remain at normal risk levels, there should be sufficient discipline of inefficient or exploitative insurers.

Guaranteed renewability in its several forms provides sufficient protection for most people who start out as normal risk. For those already at elevated risk, for instance those with genetic diseases, or those who already have some chronic condition, some public intervention will be needed. A sensible strategy would be to provide a credit towards insurance purchase which is greater for higher-risk people. The basis for this credit could either be documentation of the presence of a set of conditions which are agreed to represent high risk, or evidence that the person paid a high-risk private insurance premium. In this latter case, the credit cannot fully offset any risk-related premium, since then insurers could conspire with potential insureds to represent themselves as high risk. But it could be some proportion of any additional premium, with the level of coverage being related to the administrative costs and moral hazard issues raised above.

In short, it will not be possible to protect someone completely against the risk of becoming a high risk. One may question whether complete protection is necessarily desirable. One may also note that, if the level of coverage is a choice variable, community rating has an additional defect of inducing the purchase of too much insurance by the high risk, and too little insurance by the low risk. Somewhat paradoxically, the presence of variability in risk can either cause the very high risks or the very low risks to fail to obtain coverage.

FAIRNESS TO PROVIDERS

A recent study by Victor Fuchs indicates that, with regard to physician services, one of the differences between the USA and Canada is that physicians receive a substantially higher net income in the USA, without serious offsetting adjustments in hours or difficulty of work, but with some tilting of the special composition of the profession in Canada toward GPs and family practitioners.[9] US doctors make more because they charge and get paid more. It appears that the primary explanation of how the health care share of GNP diverged since the late 1970s between the USA and Germany is a higher rate of growth in input prices in the USA relative to Germany. And the recent real growth in hospital costs in the USA, though at about the usual trend of 6%, is more heavily composed of increases in wage rates than has historically been true.

It is notoriously difficult to determine what the right wage should be, especially for labour furnished by professionals with specialised training. In ordinary markets, the question usually is whether sellers have monopoly power—the ability to push the price above a competitive level. But in the health care market in a government-dominated system, it is clearly possible for the government, as proxy buyer, to force price below the competitive level. A lower price paid to providers depresses the quantity somewhat, but it still may benefit most consumers (those who are able to get care or those who do not happen to get sick) by lowering insurance costs sufficiently.

The main economic point to be made here is that lowering expenditures by depressing provider prices is not an unmitigated good. For one thing, lower expenditures need not mean a lower aggregate cost for the economy: consumers who are not providers sacrifice less consumption, but consumers who are providers sacrifice more consumption. On balance, the sacrifice in real consumption when providers are paid less in Canada need be no less than in the USA. It is just a matter of who does the sacrificing.

How can the price paid to a supplier of an input be pushed below the competitive level? Won't they do something else? The answer can be negative if the inputs are specialised. In the case of physicians, nurses, and other health professionals, such specialisation certainly is present. Doctors and nurses, once they are trained, have few other options. A powerful buyer can depress prices by taking away what economists call their quasi-rents—the excess of the competitive price over what a person needs to keep him or her in a job for which a specialised investment has been made.

It is not efficient to depress prices below the competitive level. It may not be fair. Balancing the health care budget by holding down nurse wages sounds unfair. Doctors have been accused, with some circumstantial evidence, of charging monopoly prices when they do not face a major buyer. But the problem is that the ability of a dominant government to push down returns does not stop when the competitive price (in this case, a price sufficient to cover their cost of education and the opportunities doctors forgo as part of training) is reached.

The problem is that we just do not know whether the price is close to the competitive one, if you would define that as fair, or whether it is above or below. What we can say is that enthusiasm for cost containment that is brought about by curbing input prices should be less than unbounded, at least compared to the alternative of controlling costs by chewing up fewer real resources.

MOVING TO EQUITY AND EFFICIENCY

If we take a bottom-up view of equity we want to make it possible for people to spend more than the minimum. Canada prohibits this: private insurance and payment in excess of government-set prices is illegal. But if we do choose a system in the USA in which it is possible to spend more, the basic system must have some devices to make sure that people do not overspend. One good way to control spending (and use) is to make expensive care cost something, rather than to make it all free. For very low-income people, those most likely to use below the minimum, we do want care to be free. But for others, who would be willing to buy more, we face a paradox. To achieve more equal use, we need to have more unequal insurance coverage. To be blunt, the minimum coverage—the coverage we want to be sure everyone has—need not and probably should not be as generous for high-income people as for low-income persons.

To be sure, if a well-to-do person wants to buy generous coverage entirely with his own money, the 'bottom-up' view would not prohibit it. But the minimum coverage, the coverage that is an object of public concern and possibly of public subsidy, need not be nearly so generous.

ACHIEVING BOTTOM-UP EQUITY IN A MARKET SYSTEM

Equity questions do not have clear answers, and Canada has answered them differently from how the USA might. I will conclude by outlining briefly the principles that I would suggest for an equitable and efficient USA system. This concept, labelled 'responsible national health insurance' is described in detail elsewhere.[10]

Briefly the scheme involves:

1. A requirement for minimum insurance coverage imposed on individuals.
2. Tax credits to make the insurance affordable.
3. The required level of coverage to be more generous at lower than at higher incomes.
4. Income and payroll tax system used to enforce requirement.

5. Credits to vary with risk level.
6. Contracted 'fallback' insurance for persons who do not obtain their own.
7. Insurance expected to be obtained through employment group for most persons.

This scheme provides equitable coverage, paid for in an equitable fashion. It is also neutral with regard to how one buys insurance, and neutral with regard to whether the person chooses, with his or her own resources, to buy coverage in excess of the minimum. It stands a good chance of being more closely attuned than the Canadian system to the desires and diversity of USA citizens.

CONCLUSION

Equity ought, in my view, to be part of any national health care policy, but it ought to take a special form in the USA, different from Canada, depending on some specific factors. If tastes are more diverse in the USA, there should be less enforced uniformity. If Americans prefer bottom-up equity to top-down equity, private supplementation of any public insurance should be made easy. The amount of financing shifted from the public to the private sector should depend on a comparison of the excess burden cost of tax finance with any administrative cost savings. There should probably be some variation in premiums with risk, depending on the strength of possible incentive effects, and public intervention to equalise premiums should depend on the ability of the private market to supply guaranteed renewability, and the feasibility of risk-related tax credits. Cutting costs by forcing providers to take less should not overshoot the competitive level. Most important of all, we need to design *unequal* insurance coverage, and use it to bring about an ability and willingness to use and pay for care that improves consumers' health.

REFERENCES

1. Rawls, J. *A Theory of Justice*. Cambridge, MA, Belknap University Press, 1971.
2. Sullivan, C. and Rice, T. The health insurance picture in 1990. *Health Affairs* 1991, **10** (Summer); 104–115.
3. Reinhardt, U. E. Health insurance for the nation's poor. *Health Affairs* 1987, **6** (Spring): 101–112.
4. Grannemann, T. Reforming national health programs for the poor. In: M. V. Pauly (ed.) *National Health Insurance: What Now, What Later, What Never?* Washington DC, American Enterprise Institute, 1980, 104–136.
5. President's Commission for the Study of Ethical Problems in Medicine and Biomedical and Behavioral Research. *Securing Access to Health Care*. Washington, DC, USA Government Printing Office, March 1983.
6. Ballard, C., Shoven, J. and Whalley, J. General equilibrium computations of the marginal welfare costs of taxes in the United States. *American Economic Review* 1985; **75(1)**: 128–138.
7. Danzon, P. *The Hidden Cost of Budget-Constrained Health Insurance Systems,* American Enterprise Institute working paper, Washington, DC, December 1991.
8. Health Insurance Association of America. *Health Care Financing for all Americans: Private Market Reform and Public Responsibility,* Washington, DC, HIAA, 1991.
9. Fuchs, V. R. and Hahn, J. S. How does Canada do it? A comparison of expenditures for physicians' services in the United States and Canada. *New England Journal of Medicine*, 1990; **323**: 884–890.
10. Pauly, M. V., Danzon, P., Felstein, P. and Hoff, J. A plan for responsible national health insurance. *Health Affairs* 1991, **10** (Spring); 5–25.

CHAPTER 4

Lessons in long-term care: the benefits of a northern exposure

Robert L. Kane
School of Public Health, University of Minnesota, Minneapolis, Minnesota, USA

INTRODUCTION

Canada stands as an important lesson for the USA. At the very minimum it represents the art of the possible. For those interested in long-term care (LTC), it suggests that it is possible to include LTC in a programme of universally accessible care without national bankruptcy. Although some of the claims that health care spending as a proportion of gross national product (GNP) may cast the Canadian situation in too favourable a light compared to the USA because of its more improved GNP, there seems to be agreement that, at a minimum, costs of health care in Canada are not rising any faster in Canada in the last quarter century despite the great increase in access to many forms of care, including LTC.[1] At the same time, universal health insurance is a vehicle to get to a solution rather than a panacea. It provides a structure through which other steps to reforming LTC can be taken, but its presence is not a guarantee that those steps will be taken.

An early word of caution is in order. Any model from

North American Health Care Policy in the 1990s
Edited by A. King, T. Hyclak, S. McMahon and R. Thornton

another society, even one culturally similar, is not necessarily importable intact into our country. Differences in basic values, such as the role of government and the centrality of the individual, must be recognised and accommodated. Nonetheless, the fact that quite different approaches are possible, and are associated with controlled costs, provides important evidence in the pressure for change.

WHERE DOES LONG-TERM CARE FIT?

Although the term implies a distinction from acute care, the concept of LTC remains somewhat elusive. In the past, it has meant that portion of chronic care provided to persons who have lost (or never obtained) the capacity for providing their own medical, personal and social needs. It has largely been thought of as care rendered in institutions like nursing homes. Indeed, the nursing home has become the touchstone of LTC, with other forms of this care referred to as 'alternatives' to nursing home care. Policy questions were posed in terms of whether other forms of care (usually care provided in the client's home or in other community-based sites) could prevent or delay admission to a nursing home. Only gradually has the policy debate begun to redefine the question to recognise that most people strongly prefer to remain at home whenever possible. Thus, community care is the primary goal of LTC, but the condition of many persons needing LTC is such that some form of institutional care may be necessary. The policy objectives then become maintaining the dependent person's functioning in the situation best suited to that task, while preserving the individual's autonomy under a general cost constraint.

With the changes in acute care, especially the push in the USA to reduce hospital use by shortening stays, there has emerged a new form of care that lies somewhere between acute care and LTC, namely services provided in what have been considered LTC situations (i.e. nursing homes and home care) but directed at patients who previously would have been cared for in a hospital.

Nor does long-term imply the absence of acute care. Persons who receive LTC do not cease to need acute care as well. Nursing home patients continue to require the regular attention of physicians to attend to their many medical problems. In fact, they are more likely than those living in the community to make use of hospitals. Thus, the distinction between acute care and LTC is, in several senses, arbitrary. It is not a case of either/or, but of how to create a system of care that can address the needs of that sector of the population with chronic medical problems, which often include social and psychological complications.

The Canadian experience is informative for what it can show about how the situation is improved when the problem of access is relieved. Once ability to pay for care is no longer a problem, other challenges remain, for example how to coordinate acute care and LTC services. Historically, LTC has been sponsored by social agencies, which do not automatically interface well with medical sponsorship. Each represents a different social construct with a language and style of its own. Several Canadian provinces have begun to confront this problem by bringing the two programmes under the same aegis, but none would claim to have solved it.

Another important issue in LTC is the role of the informal support system. This term is largely a euphemism for family, which in turn really means females. Spouses, daughters and daughters-in-law provide the bulk of LTC in both countries. Especially in the USA, there is a continuing concern that if more formal (i.e. paid) services are provided, families will reduce, or even cease, their efforts to care for their own. The experience in Canada can help to alleviate this concern. There is no evidence of any falling off in informal care despite more available formal LTC benefits. Nor has the so-called 'woodwork effect' occurred, whereby excessive demands for care are triggered by the availability of public support. Although there were early pressures placed on generous systems, these were readily managed by simple case management procedures.

OVERVIEW OF THE CANADIAN SITUATION

Before discussing the Canadian LTC situation and its possible lessons for the USA, a few basic points need to be made. The Canadian system of health care financing is essentially a provincial model. Provinces have primary responsibility for health care. Each province participates in a federal programme whereby the federal government provides a fixed-sum grant to each province to support its health care system in exchange for the province's commitment to four principles of health care: (i) universal coverage of all residents in the province; (ii) transportability of coverage across provinces; (iii) provision of at least a minimum benefits package (including both ambulatory and inpatient care, but not requiring LTC); and (iv) publicly administered programmes (i.e. private intermediaries are not permitted). To these have recently been added the proscription against extra-billing (or balance billing) by physicians. That is, physician plan members are precluded from charging their patients more than the fee schedules negotiated each year. (In American parlance, e.g. in the Medicare programme, this is equivalent to accepting assignment.) LTC is not included as a mandatory benefit nor is any special federal revenue provided to cover its costs. Nonetheless, eight of the ten provinces include some level of long-term coverage within their health programmes. Most are quite comprehensive, covering both institutional and community care.

Canada represents a quite different scale from the USA. Its entire population is less than that of California. This situation provides us with useful information about the feasible scale of operations. As discussions in the USA turn from an eye on Washington to a hopeful glance at the state capitals, the information that quite small provinces can operate an efficient system of universal health insurance with populations of less than 1 million provides some hope for those now looking to state solutions at least as innovative forerunners of a national programme.

Most Canadians live in a narrow band not far from the border with the USA. Thus Canadian provinces face the familiar problem of addressing the needs of scattered rural groups as well as urban centres.

LONG-TERM CARE ISSUES

The major lesson to be learned from the Canadian experience is that universal health insurance that includes LTC is feasible. Canadian feasibility is not universally accepted as proof of potential American success. It is true that Canadians seem to treat their government differently from Americans and are more likely to look to it to provide social services, but recent events suggest that Canada is not the haven of 'peace, order, and good government' that its founding document, the British North America Act of 1867, would suggest. Canada may be as capable of internal schisms as the USA.

Nor does the existence of a payment system for LTC solve many of the delivery and organisational problems that beset both countries. Both must contend with the existence of strongly entrenched institutional care commitments, the costs of which increase yearly as both the demand and unit costs escalate. Finding resources to encourage the growth of community-based care while attending to the demands of the institutional sector can be very difficult.

At the same time, having a single payment source allows both overt and covert redistribution. Such redistribution has been championed in the USA as well. One of the loudest cries has come from Daniel Callahan, who has suggested a dramatic policy shift away from high technology for the elderly to more support for LTC.[2,3] The reception to his proposal and to a related set of activities in Oregon, where the state is attempting to redistribute Medicaid resources away from expenditures on high technology (labelled as inefficient) to more primary care (ironically almost totally avoiding any coverage issues related to older persons), suggests the kind of reception such a proposal is likely to have in the USA. There is an immediate response of ageism and prejudice, despite a general sentiment in favour of re-examining national priorities for health care and a greater willingness to forgo heroic treatment in the period immediately prior to death.

In Canada, the provinces that introduced LTC as part of universal entitlement shifted resources from acute to chronic care to accomplish part of this inclusion. This shift was accomplished in several ways. Hospital growth was slowed. The proportion of increase going to acute care during the years following inclusion was less than in prior years, and the growth in LTC spending was much larger than that for acute care.[4] The lack of dramatic outcries from the hospital sector can be explained in part by the nature of Canadian funding for hospitals. Hospitals are paid on a global budget basis. They receive effectively a lump sum amount for the care they deliver. This amount is adjusted annually to recognise marked changes in case mix or volume. Such a payment scheme provides incentives to reduce costs of care (even more powerfully than do diagnostic related groups—DRGs). One way to lower the costs of care without affecting census is to keep patients who need only chronic care longer. Thus, a hospital may complain publicly about 'bed blockers' who are hard to discharge, but may appreciate their role in lowering the average daily cost of care.

In some provinces, the government actually required that hospitals transform a fixed proportion of their beds from acute to chronic care (called 'extended care'). This transition serves two purposes: (i) it provides a hospital-based system of LTC that should improve the overall quality; (ii) in effect, it controls hospital cost by reducing (albeit subtly) the supply of acute beds.

There is no question that Canadian provinces have been more willing to ration expensive medical technology than have Americans.[5] (Some might prefer to call it 'rational spending'.) Per capita, the USA performs almost three times as much open-heart surgery, eight times as much radiation therapy, and six times as much lithotripsy as Canada.[6] Canadians have used their single payer approach to establish regional treatment centres, where technological expertise in a given procedure is concentrated and the numbers of cases performed improves both efficiency and quality. Because they have used median figures for their planning, there is a greater risk of waiting lists than in the comparable American situation, where planning is based on providing maximal access to a perceived market and sometimes then having to create a demand to justify the supply.

The development of extended care beds in hospitals has created some problems. The boundaries between acute and chronic care are still difficult to draw. Even this complement of beds becomes quickly filled, leaving hospitals to negotiate with the community to find placements for the patients they are anxious to discharge. The community, in turn, views the hospital as both a source of patients and another provider of LTC. There is concern that the hospitals may skim the cream, sending out the most difficult cases. The duplication of effort creates problems for the administrative structure by muddying the lines of authority and responsibility. In general, the interface between hospitals and community providers has not been any smoother in Canada than in the USA.

MODELS OF LONG-TERM CARE SYSTEMS

Several provinces have taken advantage of the unified payment for LTC to develop coordinated models of services. Manitoba established one of the early provincial models with an Office of Continuing Care. This office operated what might be considered, in American terminology, a case management programme, including pre-admission screening. In effect, the emphasis is somewhat different. Clients, their families, concerned neighbours, health professionals or others can refer cases to the programme. Each client is assessed (by a team of nurse and social worker) to determine care needs and preferences. Care needs are classified into four basic levels, each of which can be theoretically met in either community or institutional settings. In practice, it is inefficient to meet the most basic needs in institutions or usually to sustain very dependent care for long periods in the community. But the principle is important: clients are evaluated on their needs independent of a decision about how to meet those needs. Clients are then given a choice of venues for care (home care or institutional care) and, within those venues (especially for institutions), a choice of providers. (For home care, there is usually less choice among agencies but choice among specific care givers.) Thus, an individual can opt to be admitted to a particular institution that serves a religious or ethnic group, or is located in a desired place. If there are no beds available in the desired institution, the client can go on the waiting list, and in the meantime either remain in the community or go to a less preferred place in the interim.

The choice of institutional versus community care is made in a fiscal situation that, if anything, favours institutional care. Home care is given without charge. Nursing home care includes a modest co-payment, established to estimate the room and board cost but, in essence, driven by the amount available to the person living on only a government pension and retaining about $125 a month for personal items. Thus, nursing home care is a good buy, and home care has no financial barriers.

Nonetheless, the 'woodwork phenomenon' so feared in the USA, whereby swarms of people will begin to demand care if cost is no longer a barrier, has not been evidenced. Although there was a brief flurry of demand for home care, especially for chore services when the programme began, this response was readily controlled by the care coordinators. With regard to nursing home care, the strong disinclination to enter such an institution is a sufficient force to prevent untoward utilisation. Most older people very much want to stay in their homes as long as possible. Indeed, they will go to great extremes, even sometimes imperil their health, to remain there. Similarly, most families continue to provide extensive care even in the presence of formal services.

With much of the activity related to managing LTC, the physician has been displaced from his central role. He is more likely to serve as a member of an interdisciplinary team than to be the final arbiter of what kinds of care are needed. Unlike the situation in the USA, physician referral is not a precondition to receiving LTC services. In the USA, both home care and nursing home admissions require a physician order. At the same time, one does not want to discourage physicians from playing an active role in ongoing care of LTC recipients. Primary care is essential to their well-being and continued functioning as independently as possible.

Canada has a stronger tradition of primary care than does the USA. A larger proportion of physicians are in primary care rather than in specialties in Canada. Perhaps not just coincidentally, the fee schedules for procedures are less likely to encourage highly technical, often expensive care. Canadian physicians earn less than their American counterparts, but the differences are especially pronounced in the payments for technically complex surgical procedures.[7] The average American payment for coronary bypass surgery or intra-ocular lens replacement is up to four times that of the Canadian average.[8]

Displacing the physician from his historical role as the authoriser of LTC services can have serious negative consequences for primary care of LTC clients. Alienating physicians will not help to assure that their patients continue to receive active primary care. Certainly entry into LTC should not be a signal that the client is disenfranchised from acute care. Quite the contrary, LTC clients are likely to need more, not less, physician attention.

The Manitoba model has an interesting component, which helps to link the medical component into the LTC system. Each case recommended for institutional care must first be reviewed by an interdisciplinary panel, which includes a geriatrician and someone from LTC as well as nursing and social work. This panel provides a second opinion, based on the report of the care coordinator. In most cases this is simply a quick affirmation of the plan, but in some instances the panel may recommend that the client receives a more comprehensive geriatric evaluation. Geriatric evaluation units have been established at the major hospitals, often in conjunction with extended-care beds. These teams can examine the patient to determine if there are remedial conditions that, properly treated, might either eliminate the need for heavy care or minimise the care burden.

Although the care coordination provides linkage between community care and institutional care at the time of determining eligibility, Manitoba has two separate systems to oversee the ongoing care. The regulation and funding of nursing homes is separate from that for community care. And each is separate from that for hospitals.

The Manitoba approach has been adopted and adapted by several other provinces, which have observed its operation and used components without necessarily buying the whole. British Columbia has an active programme of both community and institutional care. The community care is coordinated through local health departments, which contract with community agencies to provide services. In some instances, the health departments have used this contracting authority specifically to encourage quality of care. They have incorporated into the criteria for a contract evidence of quality based on consumer reports and response to referrals. Figure 4.1, taken from a 1990 report from the Vancouver Health Department, shows how the care rendered in the community is more tilted to the less impaired clients, but that even those rated as needing extended care can be served in the community. The five levels of care correspond to increasing intensity from personal care through extended care. Note also that more clients are served overall in the community than in nursing homes. The extended care described here does not include that provided in acute hospitals, which use a different administrative and information system.

The Alberta system of LTC is also heavily influenced by the Manitoba approach. This province represents an example of reverse flow. They have incorporated the case-mix reimbursement approach used by several states in their payment scheme for nursing homes. Their approach, however, uses a more detailed and sensitive method, which recognises the important distinction in determining the need for assistance with activities of daily life (ADLs) between doing the task and supervising its performance.

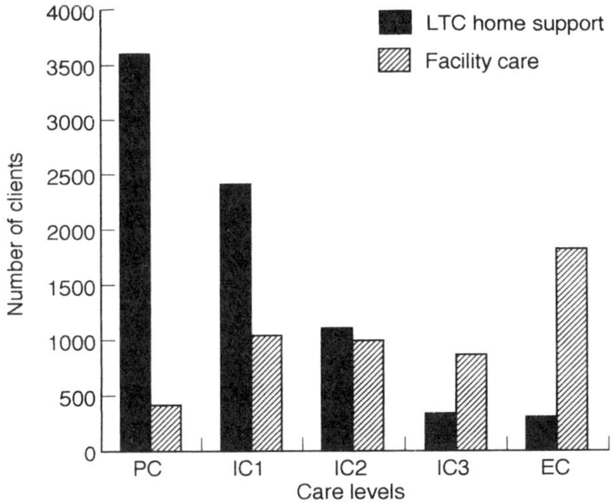

Figure 4.1 LTC home support and facility care clients by care level for 1989. (From Vancouver Health Department, Continuing Care Division, Annual Report, 1989)

Ontario has recently gone through a thorough review of its LTC and has produced a planning document that outlines dramatic reforms.[9] Up to this point Ontario had an awkward arrangement with regard to institutional care. Its supply of homes for the aged had originally been developed under the aegis of either local governments or charitable organisations. With the inclusion of coverage for LTC under the provincial medical plan, there was a strong effort to recognise many of these homes to provide nursing home care as well as residential services and hence to pay them from the provincial health plan for these services. However, the homes for the aged had historically been overseen by the Ministry of Community and Social Services, rather than Health. The ensuing situation was confusing, with duplicate administrative structures, unclear standards or responsibility, and apparent discrepancies in the rate of payment to nursing homes and homes for the aged for allegedly similar cases. At the same time, there was a general lack of activity in community-based LTC. Most of the home care services were directed at acute care to facilitate the discharge from hospitals or to serve as alternatives to hospital admissions.

The proposed changes announced in 1990 describe a more coordinated approach, which introduces a combined agency that links the two ministries to oversee and coordinate geographic responsibility to provide, in the most extreme, a fixed amount per capita to cover the costs of LTC in institutions and in the community. The plan calls for decentralisation. A single agency would be responsible for the entire programme within a region. Nursing home payment would be based on the costs of caring for different types of patients, along the lines of the case-mix reimbursement systems used in many states. Co-payments would continue for this type of care, but be linked to ability to pay. More attention and support would be shifted to community care, with efforts to consolidate and strengthen in-home care. Co-payments for household chore services would also be used (on a sliding scale).

Ontario has already committed itself to a programme of regional geriatric centres, which are intended to provide greater coordination of specialised geriatric care, including assessment, and to promote the growth of specialised services for dependent older persons.

However, the LTC reform proposal was introduced by a government that is no longer in power. It remains to be seen how much of this momentum will be retained by the new government.

The revolution in Ontario would bring it more into line with the changes that have already been introduced into Quebec. This province was one of the first to institute a policy of converting acute care beds to LTC. In 1979, they developed a programme of local community care centres responsible for geographically defined areas. These centres provide a mix of services including home health care and home care.[10] They are expected to coordinate their care with hospitals assigned to the same regions and to work with geriatric services wherever they are available. One of the thrusts in the province is to provide access to specialised geriatric services. The coordination seems to succeed to a reasonable degree, although the separate traditions of the various institutions are hard to overcome. Although the provincial government is pursuing a policy that would de-emphasise institutional care, there is still a strong nursing home component in Quebec. The desire among older persons to enter an institution seems to be driven less by functional status (i.e. the person's ability to perform the basic tasks needed to care for himself) than by the condition of current housing and the availability of assistance from children.[11]

LESSONS

A number of lessons can be drawn from the Canadian experience. The feasibility of universal coverage always comes to the top of the list. So too does the possibility of reorganisation, but it is foolish to deny the strength of the existing players and the pressures for maintenance, to say nothing of growth, from these sectors. Nonetheless, it is possible to transfer resources from acute to chronic care and from institutional to community care. The American error has been to expect that the existence of community care automatically leads to diminished demand for institutional care. It will not. For one thing, the use of institutions is hard to predict. Single variables like functional status or social support (the care and assistance provided by family and friends), even if defined and measured, do not explain a great deal by themselves. At the very least, there is likely to be an interaction, whereby social support is needed only in the presence of functional dependence. But even then, their predictive power is limited. However, the presence of adequate community care provides a political opportunity to push for a shift in funding, or at least a priority for future funding increases that moves from institutions to the community.

Community care is not necessarily cheaper. In Manitoba recently a provincial commission was appointed to look for ways to save money in community care. The continuing care programme was threatened by the findings that such care was not necessarily being efficiently delivered. Economies in the programme could be achieved with little apparent harm to its overall effectiveness, but still the costs of such care are not appreciably less than those delivered in a nursing home. If the full costs are considered, that is, factoring in the role of room and board into both, community care is usually more expensive. When case management is added, the costs of community care increase still further, depending on how elaborate is the case management structure.

There has been great concern expressed about the dangers of eroding the role of the family in providing LTC services if better organised, more accessible formal services were made available. The Canadian data help to dispel this myth that families will abandon their frail elderly members as soon as formal services were affordable. The results of several studies in Canadian provinces with well-developed community care programmes show that families continue to provide about 80% of the total care given—about the same proportion as has been reported in the USA.[12–15]

SERVICES VERSUS PENSIONS

There are at least two distinct ways to improve the lot of older disabled persons. One approach, that discussed here, is to provide them with accessible services by removing the financial barriers to care. This entails providing services at a cost that all can afford. The alternative approach is to provide older persons with sufficient pensions to allow them to purchase care if they wish. Such an approach would do nothing to address the market place for services but simply pump more money into retirement. This approach is inefficient to the extent that it provides more money for all older persons, although only some need services. It also requires high levels of individual thrift, because older persons need LTC at different stages in their lives. On the other hand, it removes from government the responsibility for assuring that needed care is provided, making it the responsibility of each individual. If that person opts to squander her or his pension on better food and shelter, there is no mandate to provide care. An intermediate position is to provide what amount to vouchers that can be spent only for LTC services. This approach removes the government from any role in shaping the delivery system and presumably absolves it of any responsibility for the care that is provided.

Some have viewed the Canadian approach to care of the elderly as emphasising services rather than money. In contrast to the USA, for example, Canada provides universal coverage for acute and chronic medical care (broadly defined) but pays lower universal pensions. The Canadian universal pension has a maximum of only $323 per month per pensioner. To this is added an earnings-related pension of approximately 25% of average earnings (with adjustments for low-income years). An income-tested supplement increases the pension to $707 per month for a single person and $1147 for a couple. The US old-age pension has no universal benefit but the vast majority of workers are eligible for Social Security, whose payments are based on previous earnings with adjustments for low-income years. The maximum amount is $899 per month for an individual and $1575 for a family. A separate means-tested programme is available as Supplementary Security Income.[16]

In 1980, American retirees fared much better than their Canadian counterparts. American pensions paid a third more of their last earnings than did Canadian pensions. The situation in Canada has improved greatly since 1980. The median income of older couples in the USA is still higher than that for Canadians (compared to the median income for all persons), but older single female Canadians are now better off than older single female Americans. At the lowest end of the distribution, older Canadians are much better off than their American cousins, because of a narrower range in incomes. Only 7% of those over 65 have incomes 50% below the median family income, compared to 22% of older Americans. This situation is relatively better for older persons than for younger people in Canada. Of those under 65, 14% have incomes less than 50% of the median income, whereas 18% of younger Americans are in this plight.[17]

The Canadian approach to paying for long-term care has been based on placing no financial barriers in the way of obtaining services and precluding the delivery of privately financed care. In essence, everyone is placed in the same lifeboat. Deductibles and co-payments are not used in acute care and are used in LTC only to displace room and board costs. In the USA there is great concern about the idea of government funds going to support those with private means. In a sense, this debate is reminiscent of the 1960s predictions of rich persons driving up in Cadillacs to receive free care under Medicare. (Those prognosticators would likely be relieved to discover that the out-of-pocket costs of care for the elderly are now at least as high as they were before the passage of Medicare.)

In the USA, the issue is very much one of whether older persons should be allowed to leave an inheritance. Observations suggest that many older persons will forgo care in an effort to leave something for their children. We may then find ourselves in the position of recommending services that the older client would not be willing to receive if she had to pay for them herself. The Canadian approach has thus far been to dissociate income and assets from receipt of services. In the USA we are not agreed on what role ability to pay should play in determining eligibility. We dislike welfare but seem attracted to means testing. There is certainly a strong faction that is reluctant to use taxes to pay for the care of persons who could pay for their own care. With regular portrayals of the elderly as wealthy, this position seems to be gaining support.

It seems equally unlikely that Americans would be as willing to remove the consumer-oriented pressures of deductibles and co-insurance. Although there is some appreciation that these forces act differentially on rich and poor persons and may cause the latter to forgo needed care, Americans distrust uncontrolled access. Either price barriers will be erected or some agency, like a case manager, will be used to deter excess use.

The Canadian approach to care is also distinguished from that in the USA in terms of the way regulators relate to their charges. Whereas the situation in the USA, especially around LTC, has become very adversarial, with providers constantly feeling that the regulators were there only to catch them out, the atmosphere in Canada is more one of shared goals and responsibilities. There seems to exist a higher level of trust and an attitude that suggests that the regulators' task is to improve care by helping the provider to do a better job, not by catching them making a mistake.

SUMMARY

The Canadian experience with long-term care provides a number of important lessons for the USA but it is certainly not a template. Whatever solutions are found for America, they will have to incorporate an American way of doing things. Nonetheless, several observations are worth making:

- It is feasible to offer a universal health benefit that includes LTC.
- The utilisation and associated costs are controllable with some form of case management. Whether or not one accepts the argument that Canadian health care is cheaper than American care, it is certainly no more expensive. The broader access to primary care services are achieved, at least in part, by less intensively available high-technology care. But the effects on health status and consumer satisfaction are at least positive.
- A monopsony approach, in which there is only one payer, provides a great deal of control over the system but it is not a guarantee that everything will go as planned.
- Paying for both medical and social services does not automatically assure that they will interface effectively.
- Government is a logical unit to organise services. Geopolitical boundaries define both responsibility and accountability. They avoid a marketing mentality driven by recruitment and selection. Government agencies need not provide all or most of the care; it can be contracted out.
- Canadian provinces range from populations of about 8 million to under half a million. Each has been able to operate

its own health care system, suggesting that a similar unit of scale would work in the USA. This suggests that states, or even some counties, could become the focus for health care.

- A block grant approach has worked in Canada to stimulate quite varied approaches to LTC.
- It may not be realistic to wait to implement a model of LTC that has been thoroughly tested. The Canadians seem willing to institute programmes because they respond to closely felt needs even though all the bugs have not been worked out. They simply couple a willingness to begin with a commitment to monitor and improve the programme as more information becomes available.

REFERENCES

1. Schieber, G. J. and Poullier, J. P. International health care expenditure trends: 1987. *Health Affairs,* 1989; **8(3)**: 169–177.
2. Callahan, D. *Setting Limits: Medical Goals in an Ageing Society,* New York, Simon and Schuster, 1987.
3. Callahan, D. *What Kind of Life: The Limits of Medical Progress,* New York, Simon and Schuster, 1990.
4. Kane, R. A. and Kane, R. L. The feasibility of universal LTC benefits: ideas from Canada. *New England Journal of Medicine,* 1985; **312**: 1357–1363.
5. Anderson, G. M., Newhouse, J. P. and Roos, L. L. Hospital care for elderly patients with diseases of the circulatory system: a comparison of hospital use in the United States and Canada. *New England Journal of Medicine,* 1989; **321(21)**: 1443–1448.
6. Rublee, D. A. Medical technology in Canada, Germany and the United States. *Health Affairs,* 1989; **8(3)**: 178–181.
7. Fuchs, V. R. and Hahn, J. S. How does Canada do it? A comparison of expenditures for physician's services in the United States and Canada. *New England Journal of Medicine,* 1990; **323(13)**: 884–890.
8. Neuschler, E. Canadian health care: the implications of public health insurance. *Research Bulletin,* Health Insurance Association of America, 1990.
9. Beer, C., Caplan, E., Morin, G. and Collins, S. *Strategies for Change: Comprehensive Reform of Ontario's Long-term Care Services.* Division of Community Health and Support Services, Ontario, 1990.

10. Beland, F. The clientele of comprehensive and traditional home care programs. *The Gerontologist*, 1986: **26(4)**: 382–388.
11. Beland, F. The decision of elderly persons to leave their homes. *The Gerontologist* 1984; **24(2)**: 179–185.
12. Chappell, N. L. Social support and the receipt of home care services. *The Gerontologist* 1985; **25(1)**: 47–54.
13. Chappell, N. L. and Havens, B. Who helps the elderly person: a discussion of informal and formal care. In: W. Peterson and J. Quadagno, (eds) *Social Bonds in Later Life*, Beverly Hills, CA, Sage, 1985.
14. Chappell, N. L. Long-term care in Canada. In E. Rathbone-McCuan and B. Havens (eds) *North American Elders*, Westport, CT, Greenwood Press, 1988.
15. Kane, R. L., Evans, J. G. and Macfadyen, D. (eds) *Improving Health in Older People: A World View*, Oxford, Oxford University Press, 1990.
16. USA Department of Health and Social Services. *Social Security programs throughout the world—1989*. Social Security Administration, Office of International Policy, Office of Research and Statistics, 1990.
17. Coder, J., Smeeding, T. M. and Torrey, B. B. The change in the economic status of the low-income elderly in three industrial countries: circa 1979–1986. In Bureau of the Census' 1990 Annual Research Conference. Arlington, VA, 1990.

CHAPTER 5

Quality assurance in Canada: what are the health professions doing?

Carol Kushner
Health Concepts Consultants,
Toronto, Ontario, Canada

INTRODUCTION

The health care community in Canada is increasingly being called upon to substantiate the quality of care it delivers. No longer content with an enumeration of its activities as a proxy measure, government funders, other third-party payers[1] and consumers themselves are demanding a higher order of evaluation. Increasingly, practitioners are being asked to prove the value of the health care services they provide.

A major source of pressure on health professionals to justify their current practices comes from funders. Since Canada's health care system is primarily supported through public funding for health insurance, provincial governments bear the brunt of increased health spending.[2] However, most of their attempts to control posts have not addressed quality of care *per se*, but rather more predictable strategies such as expenditure caps, or limits on coverage. All the same, experience with cost control both in Canada and the USA is teaching us a great deal about how the health care system works and is helping to

North American Health Care Policy in the 1990s
Edited by A. King, T. Hyclak, S. McMahon and R. Thornton

create a larger constituency for health care reform, and in particular, for quality assurance.[3]

THE ECONOMIC CONTEXT

Ever since Canada adopted nation-wide publicly funded health insurance in 1971, Canadian spending on health care—both public and private—when expressed as a proportion of gross national product (GNP), has been consistently lower than in the USA and considerably more stable (see Figure 5.1). This advantage is largely due to the administrative savings possible by having a single payer, non-profit system.[4]

Nevertheless, in Canada the proportion of provincial budgets allocated to health care is both substantial and, in many provinces, growing. For example, in Ontario, health spending in 1980–81 accounted for 29% of total provincial expenditures; a decade later it was claiming 33%, with the result that competing priorities for public funding, portfolios such as education and resource and economic development have lost ground over the same period.[5]

Even so, public support for Canada's publicly funded health care system remains very high, with virtually every poll

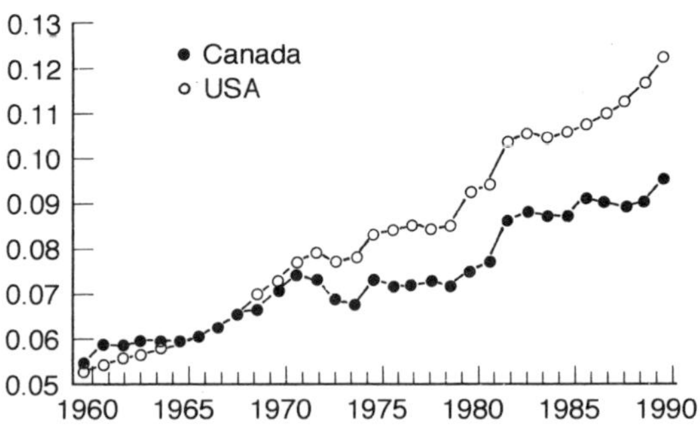

Figure 5.1 Health expenditures as a percentage of GNP in Canada and the USA 1960–1990. (From Health and Welfare Canada, Policy, Planning and Information Branch, March 1992)

indicating a preference for the Canadian system over any other alternative, including the American one.[6]

Support for the Canadian system can likely be attributed to the high degree of access to services Canadians enjoy, since under the terms of the Canada Health Act everyone is insured for necessary medical and hospital services. The terms of this legislation also stipulate first dollar coverage, meaning that no one can be charged a fee for a medically necessary insured service. By contrast, user fees, in the form of co-payments and deductibles, are the norm for those with health insurance in the USA. And even though health costs are rising in both countries, in 1989 per capita health spending in the USA was almost 40% higher than in Canada.[7] Despite these much higher expenditures, some 37 million Americans have no health insurance coverage, and it is estimated that a further 20 million are considered 'underinsured' to the extent that a major illness could prove financially disastrous to the individual. All of these factors have been well reported in our media and tend to enhance the desire of Canadians to preserve our system of publicly funded health insurance.

Recently, however, maintaining the national standards for health insurance[8] has become increasingly difficult, particularly during the current recession. The federal funding component of government spending on health care has fallen off since 50 : 50 cost sharing was abandoned in 1977. In Ontario, for example, federal contributions to publicly funded health care in 1990–91 amounted to only 34% of the total provincial health expenditures, and the formula for calculating future contributions makes further erosion a certainty.[9]

More recent federal initiatives to curb financing for health care will reduce cash transfers to the provinces to zero within the next 5–15 years, depending on the province.[10] The rapid and escalating withdrawal of direct cash funding for Medicare has forced provincial governments to make up the shortfall, since health spending in all provinces has continued to rise far in excess of inflation.

Although some provinces view these measures as an abdication of federal responsibility, not all provinces object to the federal retreat from health care. During the late 1980s and early 1990s, some provincial finance ministers began to urge Ottawa, on the basis that health care is constitutionally a provincial responsibility, to transfer all the necessary taxation power for health financing to the provincial level, leaving the provinces free to develop their own standards and their own approach to health care coverage without federal interference.

Consumer groups, many health care provider groups, and some unions fear that such a move would undermine Canada's health care system and lead to a patchwork of health coverage from one province to another. In particular, they believe that unless the federal government maintains its historical involvement in funding health care with cash as well as tax points, there will be an erosion in accessibility and universality.[11] Specifically, they worry that user fees for insured services and extra-billing by practitioners will be introduced when the federal government is no longer able to use the power of its purse to enforce Medicare's national standards.[12]

The idea that Canada ought to reintroduce what is euphemistically called 'consumer participation' in health care financing remains a stubbornly resilient one, despite excellent research evidence which clearly shows that even small user fees can deter the poor and the elderly from seeking necessary health services.[13,14]

User charges have also been singularly unsuccessful in reducing overall health care costs—if anything, they tend to be associated with higher health expenditures. In fact, the widespread imposition of user charges in the USA has been cited as a factor in the high cost of American health care.[15]

The fact that user fees do not reduce the overall amount of inappropriate servicing also tends to discredit their use as a mechanism for improving the quality of care by deterring frivolous utilisation.[16,17] However, it is the evidence of their negative impact on health status that remains the most compelling reason to reject user fees as a reasonable solution to runaway health costs.[18–21]

Since the passage of the Canada Health Act, Canadians have had protection against the imposition of user fees. This legislation authorises the federal government to withhold cash transfer payments to the provinces equal to the amount of any user fees collected.

This in fact happened during the mid-1980s, when some provinces were allowing physicians to charge patients an amount over and above the level negotiated and eligible for reimbursement by the province. In order to recapture those lost federal dollars, and in reaction to public pressure, the non-compliant provinces introduced measures to outlaw extra-billing by physicians.[23]

Prevented from passing mounting costs onto consumers, and hampered by the erosion of federal financing for health care, the provinces have subsequently resorted to a variety of efforts aimed at pure cost control. For example, British Columbia, Quebec, and now Ontario have tried to place limits on the overall expenditures for physician services. Virtually every province has tried to contain hospital expansion by restricting capital spending. Alberta has introduced changes to hospital funding linking financing to performance. More recently, some provincial governments have taken more drastic measures, opting to close hospitals despite the political cost of such decisions.[24] All of these initiatives have been criticised for their potential impact on the quality of care within our system.

Largely unexplored to date are the potential economic benefits of improving the quality of care delivered by health professionals through quality assurance programming.

FROM COSTS TO QUALITY

The assumption that *any* limitation on the provision of health care services is *a priori* a bad thing is being challenged in both Canada and in the USA.

For example, beginning with the 1974 publication of Lalonde's *A New Perspective on the Health of Canadians*[25] and with McKeown's *The Role of Medicine*[26] in 1979, there have been efforts to reassess the role and importance of health care itself as a determinant of health status. This and subsequent work has clarified that social, economic, environmental and genetic factors cumulatively are much stronger influences and are therefore potentially more fruitful territory for healthy public policy, assuming, of course, that the state has an interest in improving health status of the population as a whole.

Current efforts in Canada to refine our understanding about health status are producing new perspectives on the complex interactions among health influences and highlighting the importance of social, cultural, economic and environmental factors.[27,28] To produce the greatest positive impact on health status, it is argued that net new government spending ought to be directed towards these policy areas rather than towards health services where additional expenditures can only be expected to produce marginal benefits.[29] This position gains strength from evidence that there is a large amount of inappropriate spending on health services. Why pay more on health care, if so much of what is spent now is wastefully allocated?

Small area variation studies comparing the rates of providing various interventions in different geographical regions continue to demonstrate a disturbingly high level of clinical disagreement among practitioners. The accumulation of this kind of evidence, pioneered by Wennberg in the USA and Vayda in Canada, showing wide variation in the provision of medical services has focused our attention on the high degree of uncertainty in the practice of medicine.[30,31]

As in the USA, Canadian studies have demonstrated these variations among countries,[32] among smaller geographical regions, like counties,[33] and even among individual institutions and providers.[34,35]

Governments have concluded, and the health professions have begun to acknowledge, that in the absence of clear, unequivocal evidence from clinical research, and in the absence of explicit standards of care, wide variation in practice patterns is inevitable.[36–38]

But of course evidence of variation is not sufficient to answer questions about quality. The presence of variation merely signals the need to investigate whether areas with the highest rates are doing too many procedures, or if those with the lowest rates are doing too few. To assume that those in the middle are right could be quite incorrect. Maybe the middle-rate practitioners should be shifting their rates upwards or downwards to achieve quality.[39,40]

Research to determine whether the care being delivered is *appropriate* is absolutely essential if we are to answer these questions. And here the evidence indicates that significant proportions of care are clearly inappropriate in both high and low-rate areas. The RAND Corporation has done extensive work using research evidence and the results from consensus panels of experts to assess care retrospectively as being clearly appropriate, equivocal or clearly inappropriate. They have found that significant amounts of care are inappropriate (17% of upper gastrointestinal tract endoscopy and coronary angiography; 32% of carotid endarterectomies.)[41] Other authors report similar findings.[42,43]

Equally disturbing has been evidence that the proportion of care deemed inappropriate is *not* reduced when limits to accessing services are imposed. Blunt cost-cutting measures, such as caps on fees or reductions in coverage, may indeed decrease overall levels of service provision, but there is little to assure us that the decreased level of servicing reflects a reduction in the level of inappropriate care being delivered.

For example, in the USA a three-drug cap on the number of prescriptions for Medicare's beneficiaries in New Hampshire led to a drop in the utilisation of therapeutically important medications, such as insulin and diuretics.[44] Although it is not known whether there were individual adverse health effects because of this cap, nursing home admissions did rise in New Hampshire as compared to New Jersey, where there was no cap.[45]

As another example, the imposition of co-payments for drugs was followed by a 46% decline in the utilisation of appropriately prescribed antibiotics. Utilisation of inappropriately prescribed antibiotics fell by the same proportion.[46]

All of this evidence suggests that user fees and utilisation caps can compromise the quality of care in completely unintended ways. There is some evidence that Canada's health professionals agree, as numerous professional associations have taken positions against user fees on the basis that they restrict access to necessary services.[47]

As we develop a better understanding about the health impact of poor-quality care, the provision of an unnecessary service can no longer be seen as a neutral act. Many health care interventions carry risks, some of them substantial, even life-threatening. Improvements in decision-making by practitioners could reduce exposure to those risks, and potentially avoid additional costs associated with treating a bad outcome that may follow an unnecessary procedure.

It may be that the cost of poor quality is sufficiently imposing to shift policymakers' attention from funding issues and expend more effort on improving quality. If indeed at least 20% of all health care delivered is unnecessary, as some claim, then the potential cost savings from reducing levels of inappropriate care could be staggering. If, in addition, these savings were employed to address real but currently unmet needs, the overall efficiency of the system could be dramatically improved.

However, reducing the level of inappropriate care is not the only answer to improving quality. There is also the growing recognition that many of the problems associated with poor-quality care stem from the often arbitrary and inefficient processes involved in the provision of care. Files get mislaid, lab samples go missing, waiting times in the clinic are too long. These types of systemic problems have little to do with clinical decision-making or the skill level of an individual practitioner. Participating hospitals in the USA National Demonstration Project are finding that many times the answer lies in identifying the root cause of these kinds of quality problems and applying a systematic, data-driven approach to problem-solving known as continuous quality improvement.[48]

Consumers, too, are playing a greater role in pressuring our health care system to become more quality-conscious. What used to be a debate confined to professionals only is slowly gaining a broader audience. A recently released discussion paper about rewriting Ontario's Public Hospitals Act calls for the creation of community advisory councils as a desirable option for expanding consumer input beyond the traditional hospital board. The report also recommends mandating the publication of annual reports outlining the hospital's quality-assurance activities and its progress towards improving the quality of care and service it delivers.[49]

By and large, Canadians have been shielded from the type of information about the quality of health care services that is normally available to the American public.[50] Our newspapers do not routinely display comparative information on the quality of hospital services, nor do we yet have access to the kind of provider-specific information that is sometimes provided by third-party payers in the USA. Perhaps that is one factor behind the significantly lower litigation rates experienced by our institutions and practitioners.[51]

Nevertheless, awareness of problems with quality in the Canadian system is growing and so are opportunities for the consumer to be involved in resolving them. In Ontario and Quebec, new legislation is being introduced that will substantially increase consumer participation in, and responsibility for, the quality of care in our system.[52]

Meanwhile, the Canadian public is beginning to find out about the extent of inappropriate care in our system. For example, evidence demonstrating wide variation in Caesarian section rates in Ontario, consensus that overall rates were too high, and evidence of inappropriate provision led the government to establish a panel of providers, government policymakers and consumers to make recommendations about how to improve the appropriateness of surgical deliveries. The report of their recommendations is accompanied by a listing of the Caesarian section rates for each hospital by name. Presumably, the decision to share hospital-specific information with the public was intended to spur improvements in quality.[53] However, it is too early to say what effect this release of information will have on consumer or hospital behaviour.

Nevertheless, this approach is part of the search for levers, other than those aimed directly at cost control, to shift the focus of the health care debate away from funding and towards effectiveness.

The hope underlying these kinds of efforts is that a better quality of care will bring with it better efficiency as a desired side-effect.

There is also the possibility that a growing understanding among the public that health care is not the principal determinant of health status will produce greater scrutiny of current health spending patterns. The most optimistic view is that an increased awareness that poverty, racism and sexism are health-threatening could result in public pressure to improve health care's efficiency so as to reallocate resources to address social and economic problems in ways that could produce greater health benefits. Some have argued that a health care system with better quality would cost less, freeing resources for other health-enhancing uses.[54]

PRE-CONDITIONS FOR QUALITY IN HEALTH CARE

Despite the hope that a focus on improving quality will result in better cost control in health care, there are a number of pre-conditions necessary to actually improving the quality of care provided in our health care system.

First, we have to find out what works. Evidence from rigorous scientific evaluation about the efficacy of health interventions is an absolutely essential pre-requisite. Human beings respond with a high degree of variation to diagnostic and treatment interventions. For all but a few singularly successful interventions, only carefully-designed studies can differentiate between a good response to the treatment and a chance occurrence. Technology assessment is vital to the development of rational, evidence-based standards.

Second, we have to know the cost-effectiveness of the intervention. A marginal improvement in outcome from a therapy that is vastly more expensive than an alternative may simply not be worth the investment. Policymakers have to make choices and need reliable evidence on which to base those decisions. Those who would argue that costs should never enter the debate about quality, should recognise that the decision to devote enormous resources to marginally better technologies is also a decision not to invest in things that might produce better health outcomes. For policymakers information about cost-effectiveness is essential for making informed trade-offs.

Third, we have to have confidence in the competence of providers by ensuring that their education reflects the current state of knowledge from scientific research and that they have access to continuing opportunities to update and refresh their knowledge base.

Fourth, we have to find out whether practitioners' knowledge is reflected in their behaviour. Studies on utilisation and appropriateness are absolutely critical to identify common and special causes of variation, so that we know where to target quality-assurance efforts.

The components of high-quality health care can be summarised as having the right procedure, performed at the right time, in the right place. But of course it is also important to ensure that the procedure is executed skilfully by the most appropriate practitioner. Choosing the right thing (clinical decision-making) and doing it well (clinical competence in the execution of care) are clearly the responsibility of the health professions.

APPROACHES TO QUALITY ASSURANCE IN CANADA

Jonathan Lomas has defined quality assurance as:

> The measurement of health care activity, and the outcomes of that activity, in order to identify whether the expected objectives of the activity are being achieved, and when this is not the case, to respond with effective action to reduce the deviations from objectives.[55]

While it continues to be unclear who in Canada is ultimately responsible for the quality of care provided by our health care system, various stake-holders engage in a variety of activities related to the quality of care.

Hospitals in Canada, for example, are subject to a formal accreditation process requiring them to demonstrate compliance with a number of structural and process standards. In addition, hospitals are required to collect data on utilisation, mortality, morbidity and infection rates, and other measures associated with quality of care. The resulting hospital performance statistics are compiled by the Hospital Medical Records Institute (HMRI), a hospital-funded national, non-profit organisation.[56] In addition, all Canadian hospitals are involved in risk management activities as part of an ongoing need to address liability issues. Finally, some hospitals in Canada have begun to experiment with total quality management and continuous quality improvement—techniques borrowed from industry.

However, since the bulk of health care services in Canada are delivered in the private offices of practitioners (Canada's health care system is based on *public* insurance for *private* practice), mechanisms for delivering quality-assurance programming in ambulatory care settings are also desirable.

In 1989, the Ontario Ministry of Health sponsored a nation-wide study on the quality-assurance activities performed by the licensing agencies for five major self-regulating health professions: medicine, dentistry, nursing, pharmacy and optometry.[57]

These five professions were selected because their combined activities account for more than half of all health care spending in Canada. Provincial licensing organisations were chosen because they have some degree of authority over the professionals working in ambulatory care settings.

The results, which are based on self-report, indicated that although all 50 organisations had a formal programme for dealing with complaints about quality, only half had some form of pro-active routine audit of their practitioners. In fact, pharmacy was the only profession that had a routine audit programme in all ten provinces, and Quebec was the only province that had a routine audit programme for all five professions studied.

After a review of the literature, a framework for describing both types of programmes was developed by the researchers based on a model proposed by Dr Geoffrey Anderson and Jonathan Lomas.[58] This model involves five separate activities: define standards, collect data, assess the care provided, respond, and reassess the standards (Figure 5.2)

For each of these activities, the researchers identified the approach recommended in the literature.[59,60] For example, in an ideal world standards would be both written and explicit. They should also, whenever possible, be derived from the

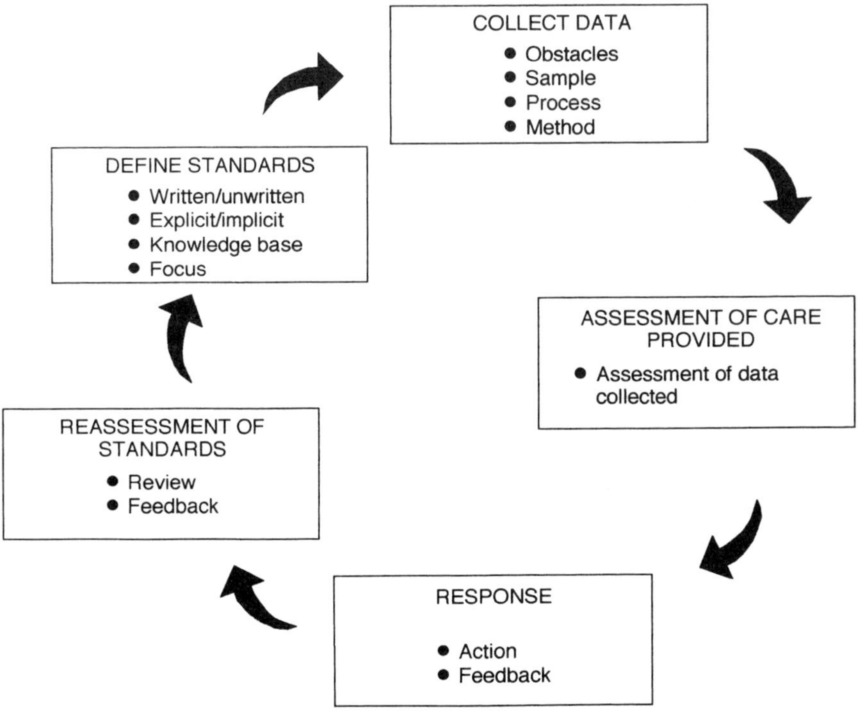

Figure 5.2 A framework for quality assurance. (From Fooks *et al.*, *Quantity Assurance in Health Care* 1990; **2**: 89–109)

current state of knowledge obtained through scientific research—a requirement that also necessitates a formal process for regularly updating the standard to incorporate new data. In addition, the focus of the standard needs to incorporate outcomes as well as structure and process measurements in order to relate, wherever possible, the quality of care to the health status of the patient.

The results revealed that although three-quarters of the 50 organisations had written standards, only just over half were considered explicit by the researchers, based on their judgement of whether or not the criteria for meeting the standard were measurable. Those organisations that had written and explicit standards were asked about the knowledge base used for their development. The vast majority (96%) reported reliance on 'usual and customary practice'. Only about one-third (38%) of the programmes incorporated a review of the literature as part of their process for developing standards.

This neglect of the literature casts doubt on the validity of the many standards of practice developed in Canada and suggests an over-reliance on 'expert opinions'. Given the extent of regional variation in the provision of services, this approach heightens the potential for competing sets of standards, as one group of experts is likely to disagree with another in the absence of good evidence.

The need for more reliable methods for diffusing scientific knowledge into clinical practice is also noted. For example, in Canada, the Society of Obstetricians and Gynaecologists has promulgated indications for Caesarian section, which were based on the literature and developed using a consensus process.[61] The resulting standard was widely accepted as valid by doctors according to a survey of practitioners, although their knowledge of its content was deficient and their rates for providing Caesarian sections were barely affected.[62]

The need to reassess standards in order to ensure that they continue to reflect current knowledge from scientific research requires a formal process. Of the 49 organisations that had developed standards for routine or complaints investigations, only three had in place a formal process for updating their standards.

This suggests a serious deficiency. Unless the growing amount of definitive research evidence is incorporated into the standards on a more or less continuous basis, the standards themselves will lose credibility within the profession, and tend to discredit the entire quality-assurance programme.

In developing a model for data collection in a quality-assurance programme for ambulatory care, it was first necessary to address some obstacles which prevented or curtailed the licensing agency from engaging in the activity. For example, of the 50 organisations in the study, 15 said that their legislative and regulatory framework did not permit them to engage in routine audit. In fact, this obstacle to routine audit may affect an even larger number of these organisations. According to a lawyer's advice on the relevant statutes and regulations, more than half (52%) may not have the necessary legal authority to conduct routine audits.[63]

In determining how to select the sample of a profession for a routine audit, the literature clearly favours a *random* process as the most likely method for obtaining a representative sample. However, in terms of maximising coverage, *cycle* selection, in which a proportion of the profession is audited each year until the entire population has undergone review, may be preferable. A *targeted* selection, in which only those groups pre-determined to have a higher likelihood of problems, is also an option. However, the latter, being explicitly non-representative, will clearly not provide information about the average practice habits of the profession overall and should be combined with one of the other methods.

The approach to data collection can vary as well. The preferred approach can be labelled as *systematic*. In this approach a practitioner's scope of practice is defined and the care provided to all the different types of patients seen is reviewed. This has the advantage of allowing comparisons of the quality of care delivered to similar patients, and of reducing the variation in judgement between assessors. An alternative approach, which the researchers called *pragmatic*, involves a random review of files with further records requested if indicated by the review of the first set. Finally, the approach to data collection can be considered *restricted*, when it is confined to the investigation of a single instance of care or the overall treatment of an individual patient, or a single type of intervention. Restricted data collection is most likely in the investigation of a complaint.

Of the 25 organisations that had routine audit programmes, 20 used the pragmatic approach, while only seven collected data using a systematic approach.

Finally the method of data collection needs to be determined. An ideal programme would include components to assess knowledge, the service provided, the performance of the practitioner, and the physical environment in which care is provided.

The majority of routine audit programmes studied, however, relied on a review of files and/or the inspection of a facility. Only 12 programmes involved the direct observation of performance, while only three involved a written or oral examination to test knowledge.

Assessing the quality of care provided requires a comparison of the data collected with the standard. The criteria used to make this assessment can be: (i) *explicit and prospective* (establishing a specific pass/fail barrier in advance of data collection); (ii) *implicit and prospective* (judging the data in terms of compliance with usual and customary practice); or (iii) *retrospective and relative* (determining the pass/fail barrier after all data are collected by applying a Bell curve to the overall performance of the group examined).

The criteria of choice (explicit and prospective) were used by only 20% of routine audit programmes and only 12% of complaints programmes.

Once the assessment is made, the quality assurance loop requires a response. Those who successfully pass the audit need to be informed, at least, if not rewarded. But the organisation also must be prepared to offer a suitable response to those who did not meet the standard.

The response following the assessment of care is probably the weakest link in the quality-assurance loop. It was certainly the most difficult to research, since most organisations did not keep clear records on minor actions, such as requiring a practitioner to take an up-grading course, or the imposition of temporary restrictions on practice. Most were only able to provide data on the most severe penalties they were able to impose: the suspension or revocation of the licence to practice.

Of the 360 000 practitioners within the five health professions studied, 172 had their licences suspended or revoked. Most of these penalties resulted from complaints investigations, not routine audits.

While it would certainly be desirable to see efforts aimed at improving the quality of care provided by the profession as a whole, all of these responses were directed at individuals. No profession was engaged in reviewing administrative data sets to determine patterns of inappropriate care across the profession, although this kind of data is used by provincial governments to assess improper billing.

Meanwhile, responding effectively to problems identified with quality remains an overwhelming challenge. Traditional techniques employed to influence practitioner behaviour include: feedback, continuing education, participation, administrative rules, financial incentives and financial penalties. John Eisenberg has noted that for medicine at least these techniques are more effective when used in combination rather than singly.[64] And while there is some evidence to suggest that well-designed programmes of continuing education can be effective in changing practitioner behaviour,[65–67] other researchers caution against concluding categorically that education alone can produce the desired results.[68–70]

THE SHIFTING FOCUS OF QUALITY ASSURANCE

As more and more emphasis is accorded to quality issues in health care, Canadians and Americans are experiencing a shift—a reorientation in the focus of quality-assurance programming (see Figure 5.3).

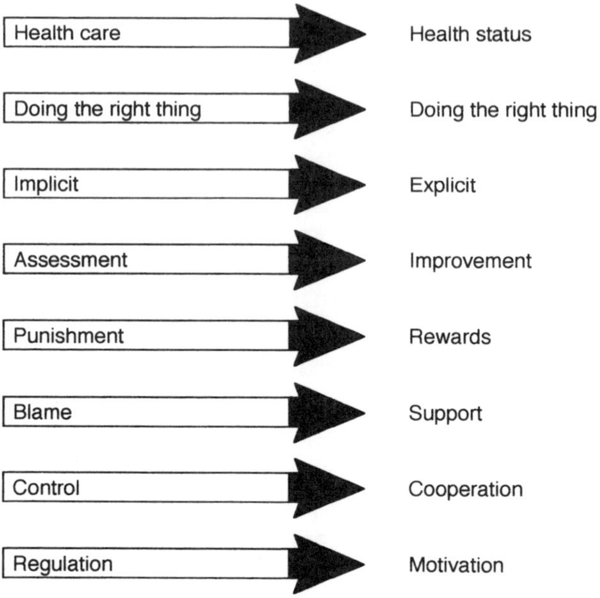

Figure 5.3 The changing focus of quality assurance (From Ontario Ministry of Health, 1990)

Aspects of this shift in perspective already referred to include more emphasis on health status as a key outcome indicator, more attention to determining whether practitioners are delivering appropriate care instead of focusing primarily on their skill in executing care, and more explicit criteria for assessing care.

A significant aspect to the shifting focus on quality assurance, however, is being inspired by a new technique for addressing quality problems—continuous quality improvement (CQI). Borrowed from Japanese and American industrial experience, CQI is based on a pro-active, data-driven, participatory approach to problem-solving which attempts to improve, on a continuous basis, everyone's performance.

While both traditional quality assurance and CQI rely on inspection, data collection and a response or action, CQI is characterised by its emphasis on the average performer, not just the outlier, and by its focus on the process and system flaws which often result in poor quality care. This reorientation—supported by data—holds great promise for taking some of the personal hurt out of quality-assurance activities.

It also appears to work—at least in non-health care settings. CQI—which is really only one component of a more comprehensive approach called total quality management (TQM)—was a key strategy in Japanese industry's rise to world prominence. But in the 1980s it has been rediscovered in North America, where it actually originated. CQI has helped Milliken Industries of Canada, a textile manufacturer, to reduce their throughput time from yarn to finished goods by 79% over a 2-year period; Milliken's on-time deliveries have gone from 97% in 1987 to 99.8% in 1990.[71]

Xerox Canada is another industry to benefit from this approach to quality. In the 1970s and early 1980s, the company saw its profits evaporate as Japanese competitors proceeded to double their market share of the copier industry. Meanwhile, experts estimated that defective products and services and failure to comply with customer requirements were costing Xerox 20–30% of its revenue. Since adopting TQM as a business strategy in 1983, customer satisfaction measures are close to 96%. Defective parts are down 73%. Harry Cogill, Director of Public Affairs for Xerox Canada, says that 'quality literally saved our company'.[72]

Only experience will help us determine whether and how these techniques can be successfully transferred to health care settings, although the early reports of the participating hospitals in the USA National Demonstration Project headed by Dr Don Berwick are providing some promising preliminary results.[73]

Much less is known about the transferability of these techniques to Canada, where competition among hospitals focuses on obtaining government funding, not on attracting 'customers' or 'market share', and where first dollar coverage removes the financial incentive for patients to select one provider over another.

In addition, little is known about how to apply CQI principles in the solo practitioner's office, where most care in Canada is delivered. Experience to date has been with large organisations like hospitals. And most of their efforts have focused on quality problems associated with non-clinical activities like portering and payroll processing.

Even less is known about how CQI principles could be applied within the context of a licensing organisation for a self-regulating health profession. Statutory obligations require licensing bodies to 'police' their membership by establishing regulations, investigating complaints and imposing penalties—none of which is compatible with the new approaches to quality favoured by proponents of CQI. Nevertheless, Berwick does believe that regulatory bodies could play a supportive role to CQI initiatives by developing sound measurement tools that represent common values; collecting and aggregating data centrally to help care givers learn from one another; providing technical support and training in quality-improvement methods; and encouraging more research on the efficacy of health care interventions.[74]

Certainly, a more cooperative, collegial and supportive ethos on the issue of quality of care is desirable. Experience from other sectors suggests that such an enormous cultural shift requires a huge investment of time, energy and commitment from the leadership of the organisations involved.

This cultural change begins with the deliberate acceptance of new assumptions about the real causes of poor quality. The most important of these is the idea that we inhabit a universe filled with flaws, and that these error-rich conditions often cause us to perform poorly despite our best intentions.

As the 'theory of flaw' would have it, most of the time problems in quality stem from flaws in the systems and processes involved in care delivery, and *not* from deficiencies in the people who are delivering the care.[75] By accepting this assessment, organisations using CQI have learned how to take the sting out of measurement and assessment, which in traditional quality assurance too often produces resentment and hurt feelings. Adopting CQI also reduces the likelihood of data-tampering, since there is no longer any reason to hide errors. Instead, the identification of a problem becomes a new opportunity for improvement. Workers become motivated to collect and analyse data about their own work processes as a way to make their work easier and more productive.

An explicit focus on internal and external customers and suppliers is also required in a culture supportive of continuous quality improvement. Thus, while the patient is clearly a customer of the physician, so is the physician a customer of the laboratory technician who receives his order for a test. Clarifying customer expectations and finding ways to meet them is central to the continuous quality improvement approach.

THE GOALS OF QUALITY-ASSURANCE PROGRAMMING

'What are we trying to achieve?' is an obvious question to be asked in assessing Canada's approach to quality assurance. Are we really trying to improve the overall quality of care delivered by health professionals? Or are we merely trying to identify, and then punish or correct the 'outlier' performance of a few individuals?

Certainly in Canada the bulk of quality-assurance programming has been dominated and limited by the latter objective. In 1989, the licensing organisations for the five health professions studied were involved in a hunt for 'bad apples' through both their complaints programmes and their routine audit practices. Most of their energies concentrated on those who were clearly outside the bounds of 'usual and customary practice'.

However, while the discovery and correction of blatant poor practice is a legitimate and necessary activity for protecting the public from harm, it is clearly inadequate to the task of ensuring overall quality of care delivered by practitioners.

Evidence of large amounts of inappropriate care makes it very dubious to assume—as we in Canada appear to have done—that the vast majority of practitioners are already providing high-quality care and that we only have to worry about a few non-compliers.

Instead, quality-assurance programming must somehow find a way to broaden its focus. It needs to shift its primary attention away from the individual 'bad apple' and towards improving the performance of the profession as a whole. It needs to encourage research that will clarify the most appropriate diagnostic and therapeutic interventions and take responsibility for ensuring that scientific evidence is reflected in practitioner behaviour. It needs to develop explicit standards of practice that incorporate patient outcome measures. It needs to be concerned that health professionals are doing the right thing as well as doing the thing right.

In addition, quality-assurance programming has to address the sources of poor quality that stem from poorly designed systems and processes. It needs to recognise that the quality of work performed by health professionals is highly dependent on the work of others, both professional and non-professional, and find ways to continuously improve the quality of overall service delivery.

Most importantly, quality-assurance efforts must find ways to become less personally threatening to the health professional. The current over-emphasis on assigning blame and punishing culprits must give way to more cooperative, supportive and productive approaches.

While Canada is only at the beginning of its exploration about how to accomplish this sweeping agenda, serious efforts at reform are being made. For example, our federal/provincial/territorial health ministers are working to establish a Canadian National Demonstration Project to explore the potential of CQI in our system. Requirements for self-regulating health professions to develop proactive quality-assurance processes are being mandated in new legislation in Ontario. Explicit standards for quality are becoming more common. Sophisticated information systems are making it possible to collect data on patient outcomes routinely. Research evidence on utilisation and appropriateness is increasing. Consumers are becoming more informed and more involved.

Together these initiatives represent real advances in Canada's effort to put quality of care higher on the public policy agenda. As economic pressures force providers to seek more cost-effective ways to deliver care, more institutions and professional associations are turning to quality assurance for solutions. Success in the long term, however, will clearly depend on the willingness of health professionals, administrators, consumers and policy-makers to participate wholeheartedly in its implementation.

REFERENCES AND NOTES

1. Private health insurance companies in Canada are permitted to sell benefits packages for services that are not publicly insured: for example, prescription drugs and dental care.
2. The federal government is less vulnerable because its contribution to health care financing is not tied to actual health care expenditures.
3. Evans, R. G. Finding the levers, finding the courage: lessons from cost containment in North America. *Journal of Health Politics, Policy and Law* 1986; **11**: 585–615.
4. Evans, R. G., Lomas, J. and Barer, M. Controlling health expenditures—the Canadian reality. *New England Journal of Medicine* 1989; **320**: 571–577.
5. Ontario Ministry of Treasury and Economics. *Supplementary Paper to the 1991 Ontario Budget: Managing Health Care Funding*, Toronto, Queen's Printer, 1991, p. 2.
6. Regular surveys conducted over the past decade by major polling firms, such as Decima Research, Environics, and Gallup, show consistently high support for Canada's Medicare system.
7. Per capita health spending (US dollars 1989, gross domestic product purchasing power parities) was $2354 in the USA compared to $1683 in Canada. (Sources: Schieber, G. J. and Poullier, J. P. International health spending: issues and trends. *Health Affairs*, Spring 1991; 106–116; and *OECD Health Data*, 1991.
8. Canada's national standards for health insurance are: universality, accessibility, portability, comprehensiveness, and public administration.
9. Federal transfers to Ontario for health in 1990–91 were about $5.3 billion; total provincial government health expenditures were $15.4 billion. (Sources: Health and Welfare Canada and the Ontario Ministry of Health).
10. In 1971, by which time all ten provinces were full participants in

Medicare, the costs of hospital and physician care were roughly shared 50 : 50 between federal and provincial levels of government, with some adjustments to provide relatively more funding to the 'have-not' provinces and relatively less to the wealthier ones.

Then in 1977, the federal government changed to a block funding arrangement which meant that the federal contribution was no longer determined by actual provincial expenditures. Future growth in the amount of federal funding for health care (and post-secondary education) was tied to growth in Canada's economy as measured by GNP.

This federal funding for health and post-secondary education comes in two forms: cash transfers and tax-point transfers. The latter refers to the transfer of taxation powers from the federal government to the provinces which occurred when the funding basis for health care switched from 50 : 50 cost sharing to block funding in 1977. Funds raised by the provinces with those transferred tax-points, however, continue to count as part of the federal contribution to health financing.

Subsequent federal budgets have made changes to the original formula used to calculate growth in federal funding for health care. In 1986, growth in block funding was tied to growth in GNP minus 2%. Then in 1990, a 2-year growth freeze was introduced. In 1991, the federal budget extended this freeze a further 3 years, after which time the growth rate for federal contributions for health care and post-secondary education will be based on GNP growth minus 3%.

It is estimated that under this revised scenario provinces will no longer receive any cash from the federal government to support health care and post-secondary education by the year 2002. This calculation is based on 1990 Conference Board of Canada forecasts of economic growth and inflation, and Statistics Canada predictions of population growth.

11. Groups such as the Canadian Health Coalition, whose members include the Canadian Council on Social Development, the National Federation of Nurses' Unions, and the Canadian Labour Congress; the Health Action Lobby (HEAL), whose members include the Canadian Medical Association, the Canadian Nurses Association, the Canadian Hospital Association and the Canadian Public Health Association are among those who want to see federal cash funding for health care retained.
12. In fact, in 1991, Quebec's Liberal government introduced a bill which would 'fine' patients $5 for the inappropriate use of hospital emergency rooms. Whether or not such a penalty would

constitute a 'user fee' under Medicare, this is an indication that the government is searching for mechanisms to instil in consumers some responsibility for their health care choices.

In the spring of 1992, a pre-budget leak indicated that Saskatchewan's NDP government was planning to reintroduce premiums for health insurance and was also considering a range of user fees for ambulance services, chiropractic services and a higher deductible for the provincial drug programme.

13. Beck, R. G. and Horne, J. Study of user charges in Saskatchewan 1968–1971. In: *User Charges for Health Services: A report of the Ontario Council of Health,* Toronto, Ontario Council of Health, 1979, 133–162.
14. Manning, W. G., Newhouse, J. P., Duan, N., Keeler, E. B., Leibowitz, A. and Marquis, M. S. Health insurance and the demand for medical care: evidence from a randomized experiment. *American Economic Review,* 1987; **77**: 251–277.
15. Schieber, G. J., Poullier, J.-P. and Greenwald, L. M. Health care systems in twenty-four countries. *Health Affairs,* Fall 1991; 22–38.
16. Siu, A. L., Sonnenberg, F. A., Manning, W. G. *et al.* Inappropriate use of hospital in a randomized trial of health insurance plans. *New England Journal of Medicine* 1986; **315**: 1259–1266.
17. Foxman, B., Valdez, R. B., Lohr, K. N., Goldberg, G. A., Newhouse, J. P. and Brook, R. H. The effect of cost sharing on the use of antibiotics in ambulatory care: results from a population-based randomized controlled trial. *Journal of Chronic Diseases* 1987; **40**: 429–437.
18. Brook, R. H., Ware, J. E., Rogers, W. H. *et al.* Does free care improve adults' health? Results from a randomized controlled trial. *New England Journal of Medicine* 1983; **309**: 1426–1434.
19. Keeler, E. B., Brook, R. H., Goldberg, G. A., Kamberg, C. J. and Newhouse, J. P. How free care reduces hypertension in the Health Insurance Experiment. *Journal of the American Medical Association* 1985; **254**: 1926–1931.
20. Lurie, N., Ward, N. B., Shapiro, M. F. and Brook, R. H. Termination from Medi-Cal—does it affect health? *New England Journal of Medicine* 1984; **311**: 480–484.
21. Lurie, N., Ward, N. B., Shapiro, M. F., Gallego, C., Vaghaiwalla, R. and Brook, R. H. Termination from Medi-Cal benefits: a follow-up study one year later. *New England Journal of Medicine* 1986; **314**: 1266–1268.
22. Mundinger, M. O. Health service funding cuts and the declining health of the poor. *New England Journal of Medicine* 1985; **313**: 44–47.
23. The mechanisms to achieve compliance varied from province to

province, with the most controversial occurring in Ontario with the introduction of legislation to ban extra-billing (Bill C-94). The Ontario Medical Association organised a month-long withdrawal of service to protest what they perceived as undue interference in physician freedom.
24. In 1992 Ontario, Saskatchewan and New Brunswick have announced hospital closures.
25. Health and Welfare Canada. *A New Perspective on the Health of Canadians* (the Lalonde Report). Ottawa, Queen's Printer, 1974.
26. McKeown, T. *The Role of Medicine: Dream, Mirage, or Nemesis?* Princeton, Princeton University Press, 1979.
27. Evans, R. G. and Stoddart, G. L. *Producing Health: Consuming Health Care*. Population Health Working Paper No. 6, Canadian Institute for Advanced Research, 1990.
28. Ontario Premier's Council on Health Strategy. *Nurturing Health: A Framework on the Determinants of Health*, Toronto, Queen's Printer, 1991.
29. Rachlis, M. and Kushner, C. *Second Opinion: What's wrong with Canada's Health Care System and How to Fix It*, Toronto, Harper and Collins, 1989.
30. Wennberg, J. and Gittelsohn, A. Variations in medical care among small areas. *Scientific American* 1982; **246**: 120–133.
31. Vayda, E. Comparison of surgical rates in Canada, and in England and Wales, *New England Journal of Medicine* 1973; **289**: 1224–1238.
32. Vayda, E., Mindell, W. R. and Rutkow, I. M. A decade of surgery in Canada, England and Wales, and the USA. *Archives of Surgery* 1982; **117**: 846–853.
33. Vayda, E., Barnsley, J. M., Mindell, W. R. and Cardillo, B. Five year study of surgical rates in Ontario's counties. *Canadian Medical Association Journal* 1984; **131**: 111–115.
34. Roos, N. P., Wennberg, J. and McPherson, K. Using Diagnosis Related Groups for studying variations in hospital admissions. *Health Care Financing* 1988; **9**: 53–62.
35. Stewart, P. J. *et al*. Diagnosis of dystocia and management with Caesarian section among primiparous women in Ottawa–Carleton. *Canadian Medical Association Journal* 1990; **142**: 459–463.
36. Eddy, D. M. Variations in physician practice: the role of uncertainty. *Health Affairs* 1984; **3**: 74–89.
37. Linton, A. L. and Peachey, D. K. Guidelines for medical practice: 1. The reasons why. *Canadian Medical Association Journal* 1990; **143**: 485–490.
38. Peachey, D. K. and Linton, A. L. Guidelines for medical practice:

2. A possible strategy. *Canadian Medical Association Journal* 1990; **143**: 629–632.
39. Wennberg, J. Which rate is right? *New England Journal of Medicine* 1986; **314**: 310–311.
40. Ontario Ministry of Health. *Report of the International Conference on Quality Assurance and Effectiveness in Health Care*, Toronto, Queen's Printer, 1990.
41. Park, R. E., Fink, A., Brook, R. H. *et al*. Physician ratings of appropriate indications for six medical and surgical procedures. *American Journal of Public Health* 1986; **76**: 766–772.
42. Chaisson, M. R., Kosecoff, J., Park, R. E. *et al*. Does inappropriate use explain geographic variations in the use of health care services: a study of three procedures. *Journal of the American Medical Association* 1987; **258**: 2533–2537.
43. Kemper, K. J. Medically inappropriate hospital use in a pediatric population. *New England Journal of Medicine* 1988; **318**: 1033–1037.
44. Soumerai, S., Avorn, J., Ross-Degnan, D. *et al*. Payment restrictions for prescription drugs under Medicaid. *New England Journal of Medicine* 1987; **317**: 550–556.
45. Soumerai, S. B., Ross-Degnan, D., Avorn, J. *et al*. Effects of medicaid drug-payment limits on admission to hospitals and nursing homes. *New England Journal of Medicine* 1991; **325**: 1072–1077.
46. Foxman, B., Valdez, R. B., Lohn, K. N. *et al*. The effect of cost sharing on the use of antibiotics in ambulatory care: results from a population based randomized controlled trial. *Journal of Chronic Diseases* 1987; **40**: 429–437.
47. For example the Canadian Nurses Association and the Canadian Medical Association both have official positions rejecting user fees.
48. Berwick, D. M. *Curing Health Care*, New York, Jossey-Bass, 1990.
49. Ministry of Health. *Into the 21st century: Ontario Public Hospitals Act Review*, Toronto, Queen's Printer of Ontario, 1992.
50. Although hospital data are routinely collected nation-wide on various measures relevant to quality (morbidity, mortality, nosocomial infection rates, etc.), the information is collected on the express understanding that its release will not identify the hospital to which it pertains. The organisation responsible for its collection (the Hospital Medical Records Institute, HMRI) is funded directly by the hospitals.
51. While litigation rates in Canada have indeed increased over the last 15 years, for physicians they are still more than six times lower than in the USA.

Malpractice insurance for physicians in Canada is provided

through a non-profit organisation called the Canadian Medical Protective Association. Their 1991 annual report actually shows an 8% decline between 1986 and 1990 in the rate of legal actions commenced. The total number of physicians in 1986 insured with CMPA was 48 618; the number of legal actions commenced was 895. Five years later 53 817 physicians were insured but only 908 legal actions were commenced.

52. Both provinces have introduced measures to increase public participation in the planning and delivery of health care. In Ontario, for example, the Regulated Health Professions Act, passed but not yet proclaimed, will require lay representatives of up to 49% on the governing councils of the licensing organisations for 25 health professions. Meanwhile, Quebec has passed a legislative package (Bill 120) which will substantially transfer spending authority for health and social services to consumers elected to boards of regional councils.
53. Ontario Ministry of Health. *Appropriate Use of Caesarian Section: Recommendations for a Quality Assurance Program,* Toronto, Queen's Printer, 1991.
54. Rachlis, M. and Kushner, C. *Second Opinion: What's wrong with Canada's Health Care System and How to Fix It,* Toronto, Harper and Collins, 1989, 223.
55. Lomas, J. Opening remarks for the International Conference on Quality Assurance and Effectiveness in Health Care, Toronto, 1989 (mimeograph).
56. The information produced by HMRI, however, is not publicly available; it is exclusively the property of the hospitals which fund the organisation.
57. Unless otherwise specified, the data that follow were taken from Fooks, C., Rachlis, M. and Kushner, C. Concepts of quality of care: national survey of five self-regulating health professions in Canada. *Quality Assurance in Health Care* 1990; **2**: 89–109.
58. Anderson, G. and Lomas, J. The development of utilisation analysis: how, why and where it's going. In: J. Lomas, and C Fooks (eds) *Conference Proceedings of the First Annual Health Policy Conference: Reviewing Utilization—The Methods and Promise of Utilization Analysis for the Canadian Health Care System,* Hamilton, McMaster University, 1988.
59. Kelly, J. V. and Keyes, M. M. (eds) *Medical Practice Patterns, Patient Outcomes and Quality of Care Assessment: A Selected Annotated Bibliography,* Association of American Medical Colleges, 1989.
60. Anderson, G. and Lomas, J., op. cit.
61. Society of Obstetricians and Gynaecologists of Canada.

Consensus Statement on indications for Caesarian section. *Canadian Medical Association Journal* 1986; **134**: 1348–1352.
62. Lomas, J., Anderson, G., Domnick-Pierre, K., Vayda, E. *et al.* Do practice guidelines guide practice? *New England Journal of Medicine* 1989; **321**: 1306–1311.
63. Ontario will be addressing this shortcoming with new legislation granting self-regulating status to 25 health professions including those studied. The Regulated Health Professions Act of Ontario requires each profession to develop processes to ensure quality of care within the profession.
64. Eisenberg, J. *Doctors, Decisions, and the Cost of Medical Care,* Ann Arbor, Health Administration Press, 1986.
65. Stein, L. S. The effectiveness of continuing medical education: eight research reports. *Journal of Medical Education* 1981; **56**: 103–109.
66. McMahon, S., McKenna, P. and Hodgins, J. An application of continuing medical education to decrease excessive lengths of stay. *Journal of Medical Education* 1988; **63**: 364–371.
67. Soumerai, S. and Avorn, J. Principles of educational outreach ('academic detailing') to improve clinical decision making. *Journal of the American Medical Association* 1990; **263**: 549–556.
68. Dunn, E. V., Martin, M. D., Bass, J., Williams, J. I., Borgiel, A. *et al.* Study of relation of continuing medical education to quality of family physicians' care. *Journal of Medical Education* 1988; **63**: 775–784.
69. Eisenberg, J., op. cit.
70. Kanouse, D. E. and Jacoby, I. When does information change practitioners' behaviour? *International Journal of Technology Assessment in Health Care* 1988; **1**: 27–33.
71. Harris, L. M. The customer prevails at Milliken Industries of Canada: eagle eye on continuing improvements, Event-Reports, Canadian Region, 1989.
72. From a presentation by Harry Cogill, Director of Public Affairs, Xerox Canada, at the Symposium on Continuous Quality Improvement in Health Care, University of Toronto, May 1991.
73. Berwick, D. M. *Curing Health Care,* New York. Jossey-Bass, 1991.
74. Berwick, D. M. Continuous quality improvement as an ideal in health care. *New England Journal of Medicine* **320**, 53–56.
75. Berwick, D. M. *New England Journal of Medicine,* op. cit.

CHAPTER 6

Management of human resources in health care: the Canadian experience

Orvill B. Adams
Principal of Curry Adams & Associates, Inc., Ottawa, Ontario, Canada

INTRODUCTION

Canada has not one but 12 health care systems. The constitution gives responsibility for the delivery of health care services for most Canadians to the ten provincial governments. The provinces' duties include 'priority setting, policy selection, planning, financing, regulating, administration, resource allocation, evaluation, standard setting and delivery of any type of health service'.[1] The federal government, however, remains directly responsible for providing health-care services to native populations (although initiatives to give responsibility to aboriginal groups are currently taking place), the armed forces and registered veterans, and provides financial support.

The Medical Care Act, which set the federal contribution at 50% of the national per capita expenditure multiplied by the number of insured persons in each province, came into force in 1968 and by 1972 all provinces were part of the programme. To be eligible for financial contributions the provinces must meet

North American Health Care Policy in the 1990s
Edited by A. King, T, Hyclak, S. McMahon and R. Thornton

five conditions or standards: portability, accessibility, public administration, comprehensiveness and universality.

By the 1970s, federal officials were increasingly unhappy about the open-ended commitment to pay half of whatever the provinces chose to spend on medical and hospital insurance, and they sought ways of gaining some control of federal spending. The result was the Established Programs Financing (EPF) Act, which took effect on 1 April 1977. (The established programmes referred to included not only medical and hospital care, but also post-secondary education, a field that does not concern us here.) This new method provided the provinces with lump sums; provinces would get the same transfer payments whether they spent more or less money on health care, and federal contributions were calculated from a base year (1975–76) escalated by the rate of growth of gross national product (GNP). The switch from shared-cost to block funding enabled the provincial governments to be flexible about how they ran their health programmes. Federal officials saw the new arrangement as giving more predictability over its health spending. (The history and development of the Canadian health care system is discussed in more detail in other articles in this series.)[2,3]

HEALTH CARE FUNDING IN CANADA

The provincial governments raise their share of revenue for health care by a variety of means, including payroll taxes, sales taxes and income tax. Of funds spent on health care in the late 1980s, approximately 42% came from provincial government revenues, approximately 30% came from federal contributions to the provinces, approximately 25% was private spending, and local government expenditures and workers' compensation schemes accounted for the remainder.

During the 1970s, non-government health spending in Canada decreased from 29.8% of total health care spending

(1970) to a low of 23.4% (1975), climbing to its present level of approximately 27%.

In recent years, total Canadian health care expenditures are estimated to be around 9.0% of the GNP. Table 6.1 presents comparative figures for Canada and the USA up to 1990, the latest year for which US–Canadian comparative data are available. In actual amounts per capita, it is estimated that the USA spent US $2425 and Canada spent US $1888 USA on health care in that year.

Health care expenditures can be divided into a number of categories. The major groupings are institutional and related services, professional services, drugs and appliances and other expenses.

The acute care hospital in Canada is the main focus of the

Table 6.1. Health care expenditures as a percentage of GNP, Canada and the USA, selected years 1960–1990

Year	Health expenditure as percentage of GNP: Canada	USA
1960	5.6	5.3
1965	6.2	6.0
1970	7.3	7.5
1975	7.5	8.6
1980	7.5	9.5
1981	7.7	9.7
1982	8.5	10.5
1983	8.8	10.5
1984	8.7	10.4
1985	8.6	10.6
1987	9.0	11.0
1989	8.9	11.6
1990	9.2	12.0

Source: National Health Expenditures in Canada, 1970–1982 and 1975–1985, Health and Welfare Canada, 1984, 1987, 1989, 1990.

health care delivery system. The ratio of total beds to population is 6.72 beds per 1000 population. There are 4.39 short-term beds and 2.33 long-term care beds per 1000 population.

Expenditures for hospitals have decreased from 44.2% of total health care spending in 1975 to 39.3% in 1988. Other institutions, especially those that treat outpatients, have increased their proportion from 9.7% in 1975 to 10.3% in 1988. The change reflects policies by governments to encourage greater use of ambulatory settings.

Physician services are the second largest component of health care expenditures, averaging 15.6% during 1978–1988. Dental services, which are predominantly privately delivered, grew from 4.8% in 1975 to a high of 5.7% in 1979 and 1980, and fluctuated between 5.3% and 5.5% for the next 8 years.

Spending for prescribed and non-prescribed drugs has increased from 8.9% of the total in 1975 to 11.6% in 1988. None of the provincial health plans offers universal first-dollar coverage for drug costs, but there is a wide variety of programmes to help special groups, notably the elderly, the indigent and those whose drug costs exceed various limits. The result is that an estimated 40% of prescription drug costs are in practice paid from public funds, and concern over rising drug costs has prompted a variety of provincial and federal studies into ways of curtailing the increases. Attempts to control the rising costs include the establishment of a formulary—a list of approved drugs and drug prices—and substitution of lower-cost drugs, especially generic copies.

Capital construction, repair and acquisitions have consumed a declining share of total expenditures as provincial governments have been increasingly stringent in their allocation of capital budgets. This has resulted in a greater reliance on capital funds from the private sector through philanthropy.

Home care programme expenditures, although still a very small part of total health care expenditures (approximately 1%), have been increasing. Over the past 10 years, provincial governments have been developing home and early-discharge programmes as an alternative to more expensive institutional care.

Provincial governments organise their systems slightly differently. This is partially reflected in differences in per capita spending across the country, which ranged from a high in Ontario of $1984.92 to a low of $1472.62 in Newfoundland in 1987.

THE HEALTH PROFESSIONS IN CANADA

The health care system in 1988 employed directly and indirectly about 7% of the total Canadian labour-force and in many communities it is the major employer. The system employs physicians, nurses, nursing assistants, occupational therapists, physiotherapists, audiologists, dentists, dental hygienists, laboratory technologists, pharmacists, radiation technologists, chiropractors and other health care providers.

Practitioners with significant self-regulatory power who 'are largely self-determining in their activities and employment' have been categorised by Lomas and Barer as 'primary' professions.[4] Within this category are physicians, dentists, pharmacists and optometrists. A second category, 'the complements', consists of health-care providers who work in a supportive capacity to the primary group; these include nurses, laboratory technicians and dental assistants. A third grouping, 'the substitutes', consists of practitioners directly capable of some of the services provided by the primary professions, for example, nurse practitioners, dental therapists. In 1992, Ontario established training programs for midwifery, a first in Canada.

Below are reviewed numbers and ratios-to-population of some of these health-care providers.

Pharmacists

Pharmacists fall into the primary professions category as members of a self-regulatory licensed profession. Although some are self-employed, most are employees of institutions

Table 6.2 Active licensed pharmacists working full-time or part-time in Canada, number and per capita 1982–1989

Year	Number	% change	Population per pharmacist	% change
1982	14 704		1680	
1983	15 337	4.3	1623	3.4
1984	15 734	2.6	1595	1.7
1985	15 957	1.4	1584	0.7
1986	16 448	3.1	1550	2.1
1987	17 009	3.4	1517	2.1
1988	17 374	2.1	1502	1.0
1989	18 337	5.5	1442	4.1

Source: Health and Welfare Canada, Health Personnel in Canada, 1991, Tables 21.2 and 21.3, pp. 126–127.

(e.g. hospitals) or retail firms. In Canada there are nine schools of pharmacy, which graduated 632 pharmacists in 1986. There has been a steady decline in the number of graduates since the high of 705 graduates in 1982.

Table 6.2 shows the number and population ratio of pharmacists from 1982 to 1989, the latter being the last year for which data are available. It shows that the growth in numbers of pharmacists has fluctuated since 1983. There have been significant increases in actual numbers of pharmacists and numbers per unit of population.

Dentists

Dentists, who also belong to a 'primary' profession, are engaged for the most part in private practice. Dental programmes are funded primarily through private insurance, although some provincial health programmes provide limited, age-specific dental care. The ratio of dentists to population in Canada has continued to increase, as Table 6.3 indicates.

The data indicate that although the number of dentists per unit of population has increased steadily during 1979–1989,

Table 6.3 Active licensed dentists working full-time or part-time in Canada, number and per capita 1979–1989

Year	Number	% change	Population per dentist	% change
1979	10 763		2222	
1980	11 095	3.1	2183	1.8
1981	11 484	3.5	2132	2.3
1982	11 880	3.4	2080	2.4
1983	12 271	3.3	2029	2.5
1984	12 624	2.9	1988	2.0
1985	13 027	3.2	1940	2.4
1986	13 164	1.1	1937	0.2
1987	13 503	2.6	1910	1.4
1988	13 742	1.8	1899	0.6
1989	13 997	1.9	1896	0.2

Source: Health and Welfare Canada, Health Personnel in Canada, 1991, Tables 7.1 and 7.2, pp. 53–54.

there has been a reduction in the rate of growth beginning in 1985. Ontario enjoyed the best ratio of dentists to population in 1988 (1 : 1697) and Newfoundland the worst (1 : 4121).

Physiotherapists and Occupational Therapists

Growth in the number of physiotherapists outstripped the growth in the population over the 1979–89 period (see Table 6.4). Despite this increase in numbers, concerns have been expressed that there are shortages of rehabilitation therapists in Canada.[5] A combination of low enrolment and low output in the universities, poor retention and high levels of part-time work is cited as the cause for an inadequate supply of rehabilitation therapists.[6]

In 1989 there were approximately half as many occupational therapists (OTs) as physiotherapists in Canada. The number of OTs per unit of population varied dramatically across the country. In 1988, Manitoba had the highest number of OTs

Table 6.4 Physiotherapists—number of active members of associations, Canada—number and per capita 1979–1989

Year	No.	% change	Population per physiotherapist	% change
1979	3945		6061	
1980	4187	6.1	5785	4.6
1981	4453	6.4	5498	5.0
1982	4536	1.9	5447	0.9
1983	4886	7.7	5095	6.5
1984	5350	9.5	4690	7.9
1985	5739	7.3	4404	6.1
1986	6039	5.2	4223	4.1
1987	6444	6.7	4003	5.2
1988	6598	2.4	3955	1.2
1989	7043	6.7	3754	5.1

Source: Health and Welfare Canada, Health Personnel in Canada, 1991, Tables 24.3 and 24.4, pp. 216–217.

relative to its population (1 : 4587). In contrast, Ontario, the province with the highest per capita health care spending, had a ratio of 1 : 10 911. Table 6.5 presents data for 1981–1989.

Registered Nurses and Registered Nursing Assistants

The number of nurses per unit of Canadian population has increased steadily during 1979–1989. Despite this favourable trend, there are high vacancy levels in Quebec, Ontario, Alberta and British Columbia. The shortages are found in metropolitan areas and in specialty nursing areas such as critical care nurses.

The ratio of population to registered nurses changed from 161 persons to one nurse in 1979 to 120 persons to one nurse in 1989 (see Table 6.6). The corresponding ratio for licensed registered nursing assistants was 308 in 1979 and 321 in 1989. Table 6.7 shows that during this period the ratio stayed relatively stable except for 1988 and 1989.

Table 6.5 Occupational therapists in Canada, number employed and per capita 1981–1989

Year	Number	% change	Population per occupational therapist	% change
1981	1852		13 220	
1982	1962	5.9	12 592	4.8
1983	2144	9.3	11 612	7.8
1984	2311	7.8	10 857	6.5
1985	2463	6.6	10 261	5.5
1986	2562	4.0	9 953	3.0
1987	2974	16.1	8 674	12.9
1988	3322	11.7	7 855	9.4
1989	3447	3.8	7 671	2.3

Source: Health and Welfare Canada, Health Personnel in Canada, 1991, Tables 16.1 and 16.2, pp. 146–147.

Table 6.6 Number of employed registered nurses, Canada, 1979–1989

Year	Number	% change	Population per nurse	% change
1979	148 954		161	
1980	155 309	4.3	156	3.1
1981	161 269	3.8	152	2.6
1982	164 231	1.8	150	1.3
1983	176 768	7.6	141	6.0
1984	188 074	6.4	133	5.7
1985	194 519	3.4	130	2.3
1986	204 723	5.2	125	3.9
1987	210 128	3.0	122	2.4
1988	210 620	0.1	124	1.6
1989	210 999	0.2	120	3.2

Source: Health and Welfare Canada, Health Personnel in Canada, 1991, Tables 14.4 and 14.5, pp. 124–125.

Table 6.7 Number of licensed registered nursing assistants—Canada, 1979–1989

Year	Number	% change	Population per registered nursing assistant	% change
1979	77 603		308	
1980	80 297	3.5	302	1.9
1981	80 954	0.8	302	–
1982	81 310	0.4	304	0.7
1983	83 539	2.7	298	1.9
1984	83 050	0.6	302	1.3
1985	83 063	0.02	304	0.7
1986	82 608	0.5	309	1.6
1987	83 610	1.2	309	–
1988	82 826	0.9	315	1.9
1989	82 281	0.7	321	1.9

Source: Health and Welfare Canada, Health Personnel in Canada, 1991, Tables 15.1 and 15.2, pp. 138–139.

Physician Supply

Physicians are the central element in the Canadian health care system. After institutional expenditures they account for the second largest component. Applegate and Garg *et al.* estimate that physicians influence or control 66–80% of health care expenditures.[7,8] They are said to have direct control on how to treat a patient, when and for how long to hospitalise a patient, which diagnostic tests and procedures to order and which drugs and therapeutic options to prescribe.[9,10] It is further argued that physicians influence the use of human and technical resources that are complementary to the clinical decisions they make.

Physician supply has grown faster than the growth in the general population. Table 6.8 presents comparative physician and population data.

The data show that the total Canadian active civilian physician population in 1989 was 51 314; of these, 52.9% were general or family practitioners and 47.1% were specialists. The year 1990 was the first since 1975 in which the population growth was greater than the growth in the physician supply. Data supplied by the Canadian Post-MD Education Registry show that as of 1 November 1990 there were 7739 filled post-MD trainee positions in the country. Approximately 83.4% of these positions were funded by provincial governments. The other positions were funded by charitable organisations and by foreign governments. Of these 7739 positions, 83.7% were filled by Canadian citizens, 6.0% by landed immigrants and 10.3% by residents of other countries.

Enrolment in Canadian faculties of medicine peaked in 1982–83 at 7492 students. In 1989–90 there were 7072 enrolees—the lowest level of the decade—a 5.7% reduction since 1982–83. It is estimated that in recent years there have

Table 6.8 Comparative rates of growth in the number of active civilian physicians and the general population in Canada, 1975–1990 (excluding interns and residents)

Year	General population	% increase	Physician population	% increase
1975	22 923 000		32 561	
1976	23 111 000	1.16	33 754	3.66
1977	23 343 000	1.17	34 860	3.27
1978	23 548 400	0.88	35 433	1.64
1979	23 907 264	1.16	36 444	2.85
1980	24 236 550	1.38	37 287	2.31
1981	24 518 400	1.16	38 310	2.74
1982	24 770 058	1.02	40 081	4.62
1983	25 029 760	1.05	41 440	3.40
1984	25 270 400	0.96	42 400	2.31
1985	25 520 710	0.99	44 230	4.14
1986	25 761 175	1.00	45 595	2.99
1987	25 784 024	0.10	47 572	4.16
1988	25 909 200	0.49	49 706	4.34
1989	26 240 000	1.28	51 314	3.23
1990	26 832 700	2.26	51 841	1.02

Source: Department of National Health and Welfare, Health Personnel in Canada, 1986, and the Health Information Division, Policy, Communications and Information Branch, Department of National Health and Welfare, 1991.

been about four times as many applicants as there have been available positions. Graduates of foreign medical schools have traditionally augmented the supply of physicians. Immigration is a federal responsibility, but provincial governments are involved in decisions permitting physicians to enter Canada. A large proportion of immigrant physicians practise in areas designated as underserviced or in specialties that are in short supply.

The federal and provincial governments agreed in 1975 to restrict immigration and the number of physicians entering as regular immigrants was reduced (see Table 6.9). During

Table 6.9 Physician immigrants and emigrants, Canada, 1973–1990

Year	Number of physicians[a] Immigrants	Emigrants
1973	1170	
1974	1090	282
1975	806	242
1976	401	363
1977	312	549
1981	382	372
1982	462	450
1983	352	371
1984	337	418
1985	342	386
1986	417	313
1987	426	387
1988	335	377
1989	459	384
1990	445	478

Source: Immigration figures: Employment and immigration Canada. (Note: not all officially admitted physicians enter medical practice in Canada. Alternatively, official immigration statistics may exclude some graduates of foreign medical schools who declare an intended occupation other than medicine but who eventually practise medicine in Canada.) Emigration figures: Sales/Marketing Systems, Southam Communications Ltd. Figures represent active civilian physicians who moved abroad, excluding interns and residents.

[a] Data on emigration in 1973 and emigration and immigration in 1978–1980 are missing.

1962–1968, the number of physicians entering Canada averaged 880 per year, representing 4.8% of the total supply. The average annual figure for 1969–75 was 1072. In 1976–1980 the number of immigrant physicians fell dramatically, averaging 331 per year. A total of 417 and 426 physicians entered Canada in 1986 and 1987 respectively, of whom 140 in 1986 and 144 in 1987 were 'selected' physicians, recruited for their particular expertise. More recent data for 1988, 1989 and 1990 indicate that there was a fall in immigration in 1988. This increased, however, to 459 in 1989, falling slightly to 445 in 1990. At the moment, Canadian immigration policy severely restricts entry of physicians from foreign countries unless they are accepted as refugees or are selected for expertise that is in short supply.[11]

The number of physicians who moved abroad in 1990 (the last year for which data are available) is 478. However, the number of active civilian physicians returning from abroad to work in Canada was 271 in the same year. Canada loses a very small number of physicians to other countries.

Activity profile of Canadian physicians

A survey in 1986 by the Canadian Medical Association of physicians indicated that approximately 89.5% of practising physicians were in full-time practice. Furthermore, 14.1% of this group were female, compared to 16.6% of the total active civilian physician population.[12] This proportion is expected to increase substantially in the next 10 years. Of the cohort of post-MD trainees expected to complete their training in 1990, 38% were female, and this figure was expected to increase to 40% in 1991. It appears that the trend will continue. In 1989–90, 43.7% of medical undergraduates in the last year, and 43.1% of first-year enrolees were females.

The effect of these changing demographics on the organisation of medical practice and the delivery of medical care is a key element in questions about future physician requirements.

Distribution of physicians

The distribution of physicians varies significantly across the country as measured by physician–population ratios. Excluding the Yukon and Northwest Territories, the ratio ranges from a high of 1:487 in Quebec to a low of 1:743 in New Brunswick. The Canadian average in 1990 was 1:518 (see Table 6.10). Comparative data for 1987 shown in Table 6.11 indicate that the ratio of practicing physicians (including interns and residents) varies significantly across 21 selected countries. With a ratio of one physician for every 464 persons, Canada ranks 11th. No relationship is apparent between the method of health care financing and the ratios. The USA, for example, with a predominantly private system, ranks ninth; the UK, with a predominantly public system, ranks 20th; and Sweden, also with a public system, ranks sixth.

Table 6.10 Population per active civilian physician, Canada, by province, 31 December 1990

Province	Population per active civilian physician
Newfoundland	614
Prince Edward Island	734
Nova Scotia	513
New Brunswick	743
Quebec	487
Ontario	497
Manitoba	559
Saskatchewan	660
Alberta	594
British Columbia	492
Yukon	679
Northwest Territories	1174
Canada	518

Sources: Supply and Distribution of Physicians in Canada, 1990, Health Information Division, Health Policy and Information Directorate, Policy, Planning and Information Branch, Department of National Health and Welfare, Ottawa, 1991.

Table 6.11 Practising physicians, population–physician ratio by selected countries, 1987

Country	Population per physician	Rank
Australia[a]	489	12
Austria	522	13
Belgium	311	1
Canada	464	11
Denmark	390	4
Finland	528	14
France	401	7
Germany	356	2
Iceland	370	3
Ireland	708	19
Italy	897	21
Japan	638	17
Luxembourg	559	15
Netherlands	424	8
New Zealand	574	16
Norway	441	10
Portugal	390	4
Sweden	400	6
Switzerland	665	18
UK	729	20
USA	426	9

[a] 1986.
Source: Organization for Economic Cooperation and Development Health Data File, 1989.

Maldistribution of physicians continues to be a problem in Canada. Across the country, governments are increasingly offering incentive and education programmes in an attempt to attract physicians to areas they describe as under-doctored. Maldistribution does not necessarily translate into reduced access to medical services; nonetheless there are a number of programmes directed to the question. The rapid growth of the number of physicians in the 1970s has not markedly contributed to improving access in rural or remote areas. Contandriopoulos and Fournier, in a study of access to medical services in remote regions of Quebec, concluded that equitable access to medical services for Quebecers as a whole was not guaranteed by the increased number of physicians.[13]

The study, recognising that physician population ratios do not differentiate between the type of physician delivering the service or the population consuming the service, developed a population services ratio. The measure was intended to indicate more accurately the differences in services utilised per capita by region by controlling for mobility across regions by physician and consumer, age, sex factors and variations in physicians' workload.

The study concluded that equity continues to be a problem in Quebec. However, the regional disparities are less when the service utilisation ratio is employed. General practice services were found to be more or less equitably distributed, although this was not the case with specialist services.

PROFESSIONAL GOVERNANCE

Lomas and Barer describe the environment that existed in Canada before the introduction of comprehensive health care programmes as one in which health care professionals practised as self-employed individuals in scattered locations with no third party intruding on the direct relationship between practitioner and patient.[4] Each of the primary professions defined the scope of its practice and controlled the qualifications of those who wished to enter the profession. The education process and the licensure requirements were controlled by each of the primary professions. The task of ensuring the competence of the individual and the quality of care delivered by the practitioner was delegated to the profession because neither government nor patient had knowledge that was adequate to judge the competence of the provider and the quality of care provided. The government established self-regulatory agencies to act as the agent of the government in protecting the public interest. Lomas and Barer argue strongly that governments, by awarding self-regulation to the professions, significantly influence the roles and relationships between health and the care providers. This has led to exclusive domains, a lack of communication between professional groups and, especially in the case of physicians, an emphasis on the individual patient rather than the population for whom they provide service.

In the case of physicians, each province now has a College of Physicians and Surgeons, which receives its mandate from the Medical Care Act of that province. The College is responsible for licensure, ensuring competence and discipline. The Colleges of Physicians and Surgeons have been reluctant to enter into questions of practice standards, utilisation of health care services and auditing of practice patterns. A study by Fooks *et al.* of five self-regulating professions—medicine, dentistry, pharmacy, nursing and optometry—found that only pharmacy in all provinces had routine audit programmes.[14] The authors concluded that the mechanisms for assessing the quality of care provided by practitioners and used by the five self-regulating health professions in Canada are at an early and unsophisticated stage, focusing only on identifying poor performers. Increased emphasis in the Canadian health care system on improvement in quality and appropriate resource allocation is putting increased pressure on self-regulating professions to be more thorough in their assessment of the competence of their members and in their patterns of practice.

Lomas and Barer suggest governments may have missed an opportunity to impose organisational change and reform health manpower roles when national health insurance was introduced between 1970 and 1971.[4] They suggest that as governments increased their responsibility for the financing of the health care system they should also have increased their responsibility for the governance of the health professions. Governments would therefore have been in a position to facilitate the use of less costly health care professionals to deliver services as appropriate. One example they cite of such a government initiative is a 1974 dental care programme for schoolchildren in Saskatchewan. That program used dental nurses or dental therapists instead of dentists.

HEALTH HUMAN RESOURCE PLANNING IN CANADA

The medical profession has been the subject of more attention in respect of resource planning than any other health care profession in Canada. In 1964 the Royal Commission on Health Services recommended increasing the number of Canadian-trained physicians, building new medical schools and recruiting foreign physicians. This recommendation was based on an assumption of growth for the Canadian population that was, in fact, not fulfilled. Between 1964 and 1973 the total physician supply in Canada increased by as much as 20%, and the number of medical schools increased from 12 to 16.

The federal and provincial governments established an Advisory Committee on Health Manpower in 1972 'to improve and maintain the supply, quality, distribution and productivity of all manpower in Canada at a level that makes possible the delivery of effective and efficient total health services'.[15] To address physician resource planning specifically, a National Committee on Physician Manpower was established by the Department of National Health and Welfare and several national medical organisations to cooperate with governments and voluntary groups in 1972. Two years later, in 1974, after the provincial Ministers of Health expressed concern about rising physician supply, the National Committee on Physician Manpower established a working group, known as the Requirements Committee, to establish physician resource requirements in the various specialties of medicine. The remainder of the 1970s evidenced a number of provincial manpower studies using primarily physician–population ratios as their base for identifying physician requirements.

A 1989 report on Canadian physician resources presents the view that the policy framework within which physician resource planning was taking place changed with the report by Lalonde, *A New Perspective on the Health Care of Canadians.*[16] Lalonde suggested that the way to improve the health of the population was not through increased emphasis on medical treatment but rather on health promotion and disease prevention. The resultant premise was that as a population became healthier there would be a need for fewer physicians in the future. Manpower planning efforts to this time had not considered the appropriateness of the services being delivered or the fact that there were alternative providers who were capable of performing some physician activities at less costly rates.

A report by Justice Hall suggested that physician oversupply be considered a primary problem.[17] This report sparked a number of provincial studies that resulted in recommendations that medical school enrolment be cut back as a way of controlling physician supply. Provincial governments began to equate the increase in physician supply with an increase in the number of services being delivered and thereby an increase in the overall cost of health care services.

In 1985, the Federal–Provincial–Territorial Advisory Committee on Health Manpower reported on the first Canadian study to include adjustments for an increasing population and a changing age/sex mix as well as changes in the physician–population mix as elements of a physician resource plan. The report recommended that a reduction in supply be effected by reductions in physician immigration, postgraduate training and medical school places—the last by approximately 17%. The report suggested that if supply continued to increase, by the year 2000 there would be a 12% surplus of physicians in Canada. The recommendations of the report were rejected by the medical establishment.

Two distinct planning approaches for physician resource planning in Canada can be identified. The first, the supply projection approach, relies on physician–population ratios and takes into account health care services currently delivered by the total pool of practising physicians. A physician–population ratio is set based on judgements about the existing level and quality of care. This ratio is then used to determine needs for physician training or immigration based on projected demand. This approach assumes that future requirements for physicians will need to match the quantity of services currently provided on a per capita basis. Possible changes in demographic features and the delivery system are sometimes factored into the projections.

The second is the demand approach, which examines the quantity of health care services demanded by the population. Physician requirements are estimated based on the number and type of projected services. Most often, this approach assumes that physicians are required for all health services that are demanded, but the approach can be modified to reflect potential changes to the delivery system.[18] Both these methods implicitly assume that the way health care services have been provided has been appropriate and that those practitioners providing those services have been the appropriate practitioners. This latter premise is being seriously questioned as the supply of physicians, the services they deliver and their costs continue to increase. Health care analysts and governments are all questioning the efficacy and effectiveness of medical treatments.

Partially in response, a third approach to physician resource planning is gaining favour within the Canadian health care system—the needs-based approach, which involves what Anderson *et al.* describe as defining and predicting health care deficits with appropriate health care services.[19] This planning method combines information on the health status of the population with disease prevalence, demographics and appropriate standards of care, both present and future. The needs-based approach emphasises services necessary to keep the population healthy. It then poses the question: which health care professional or group of professionals can provide the necessary services most cost-effectively and efficiently?

There are many groups involved in physician resource planning in Canada. The groups can be found at the federal, provincial and local levels. They are governmental and non-governmental in nature. One of the continuing problems within the Canadian health care system is the lack of cooperation between the many groups that are involved in physician resource planning. Table 6.12 identifies a number of the groups and the different levels at which they are involved.

Table 6.12 Major actors in Canadian physician resource planning

Level	Actors: Non-governmental	Actors: Governmental actors/departments
1. Federal/ national	• Royal College of Physicians and Surgeons • National specialty societies • College of Family Physicians of Canada • Corp professionnelle des médecins du Québec • Canadian Medical Association • Association of Canadian Medical Colleges • Canadian Hospital Association • Canadian Association of Interns and Residents • Canadian Association of Teaching Hospitals	• Health and Welfare • Employment and Immigration • Federal Committees • Federal/Provincial/Territorial Advisory Committee on Health Human Resources • National Committee on Physician Manpower
2. Provincial	• Provincial medical associations • Provincial licensing bodies • Medical schools	• Provincial Ministries • Ministry of Health (general funding) • Colleges and universities (education/ teaching funding) • Energy, Mines and Resources (specific programmes) • Labour, Workers' Compensation Board programmes
3. Local/ regional	• Universities • Medical schools • Hospitals	• Regional, district health councils

PRESSURES WITHIN THE CANADIAN HEALTH-CARE SYSTEM

The Canadian health care system, like other systems, is under intense review. Thus, between 1988 and 1992, senior governmental task forces or commissions were at work studying the whole or aspects of the system in nine of the ten provinces. The system is faced with the challenge of achieving a better balance between the traditional curative and institutional-oriented approach and an approach that places greater emphasis on de-institutionalisation, health promotion and disease prevention. The pressures of an open-ended, state-funded system with increasing provider and consumer expectations at a time of fiscal restraint increases the urgency of reaching that balance. The diffusion of medical technology has been carefully controlled in the Canadian system. There are mounting pressures, however, to relax these controls as queues lengthen and the turn-around time for certain medical procedures continues to be high. Also, as technology advances we are faced with a series of ethical, moral, legal and economic questions. Technologies such as surrogate motherhood and *in vitro* fertilisation and other biomedical advances make it possible to do things we thought were impossible just a few years ago.[20] There is also pressure within the Canadian health care system to reduce health inequalities, which show up, for instance, in differences in life expectancy—there remains a 5-year gap in life expectancy between rich and poor women and a 10-year gap for men.

Angus identifies chronicity as another issue. He suggests that the Canadian system has developed with a focus on the acute treatment of catastrophic illness. But today, nearly 90% of patient contacts with the health care system are for the management of chronic conditions, that is, patients who are living with a disease or disability and who need regular access to health care.

TOWARDS A NEW PLANNING APPROACH

The task forces and royal commissions that have been examining the Canadian health care system in each of the provinces have begun to consider a combination of decentralisation, regionalisation of health care services and a greater shift to community-based and non-institutional care as a way of addressing increasing health care costs. This will require the reduction of acute-care hospital beds and the development of incentive programmes for hospitals to become more efficient. It will also require an increase in the number of outpatient clinics as well as home care and community-support programmes. These strategies are to be achieved through reallocation of existing resources, not through new funds.

Other proposals are that a more efficient, cost-effective use be made of nursing staff and other health care professionals within the system. An expanded role is suggested for nurses, and their involvement in the planning and operating of all services, programmes and facilities is suggested.

The recommendations that will more directly affect the planning of human resources in health care, however, are those about the reorganisation of the health care system. These suggest that planning be at the provincial level and that specific shared goals, targets and strategies should be developed. Furthermore, in approaches to the delivery of primary health care, greater interdisciplinary cooperation is encouraged. It is also suggested that the population should begin to take greater responsibility for its own health as greater emphasis is placed on health promotion and disease prevention. Also, community-based approaches with different types of reimbursement mechanisms are being developed. Other specific organisational recommendations include establishment of physician practice guidelines, delegation of functions from physicians to nurses, development of mixed reimbursement systems for physicians and definition and clarification of institutional roles. Further, a need was recognised to accommodate additional occupational groups—midwives, for example—in the institutional setting, with appropriate changes in provincial legislation to allow this to take place.[21]

NATIONAL HEALTH INSURANCE IN PHYSICIAN RESOURCE PLANNING

The report of the 1964 Royal Commission on Health Services, which served as a base for Canada's national health care insurance system, recommended that fees for service be maintained as the basic method of paying physicians within the health care system. It recognised however, that there were other methods that would be applicable in many situations. Lomas and Barer argue that, by entrenching fee-for-service physician remuneration, universal medical insurance created 'a disincentive to the delegation of responsibility to individuals requiring less extensive training.'[4] The growth of other methods of remuneration for physicians has been slow. It is currently estimated that between 25% and 30% of Canadian physicians receive all or part of their remuneration by methods other than fee-for-service. Although the implementation of national health insurance in Canada provided the opportunity for a coordinated approach to human resource planning in health care, the fact that governments chose to act only as payer resulted in ad hoc planning approaches. Governments are now attempting to take a much more direct role here. Governments are no longer willing just to pay the bills, particularly in the face of a shrinking economy. They are now more actively re-examining the autonomy and jurisdictional rights of the health professions; indeed the roles of health professionals are being challenged from several directions at once. The challenges include the nature of chronic disease and technology innovation, but they also come from consumers, governments and other professionals—from traditional practitioners as well as from alternative practitioners. Thus, members of the health professions are compelled to recognise that their roles are changing as the health care system changes.

The physician resource issue continues to be the predominant policy question in the deployment of human resources in health care. The Conference of Federal, Provincial and Territorial Deputy Ministers of Health in 1990 commissioned a study by Barer and Stoddart. Their report, Toward Integrated Medical Resource Policies for Canada, through stakeholder analysis, international research and analysis of Canadian studies, brought forward a set of wide-ranging recommendations.[22] The researchers employ a medical career life cycle analytical framework as a method of examining medical resource policies. They point to the complexities of medical resource planning, emphasising that policies must be interdependent. Of the 11 themes presented, the following four have been identified as key:

- There is no agreed-upon policy objective for the management of the physician resource sector in Canada. The researchers suggest that the objective should be to meet those health needs of the population that can be most efficiently met by individuals with MD training. Moreover, policies in this area should be determined by the resources that society is willing to commit to meeting those needs.
- The optimal number of physicians cannot be defined by purely technical methods. Ultimately, it is social judgement, not technical judgement, that must be used. If we do not recognise and accept this, there will be unnecessary delays in the development of policy while the parties involved await improvements in data collection or planning methodologies.
- The authors suggest that a national strategy with rigid specific policies to which all provinces and territories must adhere is not feasible. What may well be feasible is a national strategy built upon the coordination of commonly understood policy objectives. Clearly, stake-holders will not necessarily all agree on all issues; also, the nature and severity of problems will vary across the country.

Nevertheless, this should not hinder the development of a coordinated approach.

- There is a need to align more closely the private interests of physicians in their decision-making process with social interests and collective goals.

The authors also deal with undergraduate medical education (suggesting a reduction of approximately 10% to maintain the current physician–population ratio), graduates of foreign medical schools and questions of licensure and training.

The impact of remuneration methods on clinical teaching, geographic distribution and specialty distribution is also discussed. The investigators suggest a more expanded approach, including not only providers and governments, but also consumers, to the development of policies. They therefore recommend improvements in the creation and dissemination of information to the public and providers.

CONCLUSION

Unlike many other countries, Canada does not have a system of public health care, but one of public health care insurance, the services being provided largely by the private sector. The system is on the whole popular with providers and consumers.

Governments, finding themselves in the position of paymaster, naturally seek to control expenditures without reducing services to the public. To this end, they have continually supported studies on the way in which resources are deployed within the system. The management of human resources has emerged as a key element in these studies.

REFERENCES

1. Sutherland, R. and Fulton, J. *Health Care in Canada—A Description and Analysis of Canadian Health Services*, Ottawa, MOM Printing 1988.

2. Naylor, C. D. The Canadian health care system: a model for America to emulate? *Health Economics* 1992; **1(1)**: 19–37.
3. Kushner, C. Quality assurance in Canada: what are the health professions doing? *Health Economics* 1992; **1(2)**, 115–129.
4. Lomas, J. and Barer, M. And who shall represent the public interest: the legacy of Canadian health manpower policy. In: R. Evans, and G. Stoddart (eds), *Medicare at Maturity*, Calgary, University of Calgary Press, 1986.
5. Canadian Medical Association, Brief to the Senate Committee on Science, Technology and Social Affairs on accessibility to acute care hospital services, January, 1990.
6. Health Manpower Research Unit—Proceedings of the workshop on priorities in health human resources research in Canada. University of British Columbia, Vancouver, 1990.
7. Applegate, W. B. *et al*. Impact of a cost-containment educational program on house staff ambulatory clinic charges. *Medical Care* 1983; **21**: 486–496
8. Garg, M. L., Werner, M., Kleinberg. Cost containment. *Medical Teacher* 1980; **2**: 222–228.
9. Komaroff, A. L. The doctor, the hospital, and the definition of proper medical practice. President's Commission for the Study of Ethical Problems in Medicine and Biomedical and Behavioural Research. Securing access to health care, Vol. 3, Washington: US Government Printing Office, 1983).
10. McPhee, S. J. and Schroeder, Steven A. The costs and risks of medical care: an annotated bibliography for clinicians and educators. *Western Journal of Medicine* 1982; **137**: 145–161.
11. Canadian Medical Association. Canadian physician resources—Report of the Committee on Physician Resources, Canadian Medical Association 1989: **24**.
12. Adams, O. Canada's doctors: who they are and what they do: lessons from the CMA's 1986 manpower survey. *Canadian Medical Association Journal* 1989; **140**: 212–217.
13. Contandriopoulos, A-P. and Fourier, M. A. Access to medical services in remote regions: myth and reality. GRIS, Faculty of Medicine. *Physician Manpower in Canada: Proceedings of the First and Second Annual ACMC Physician Manpower Conference*, 1987.
14. Fooks, C., Rachlis, M. and Kushner, C. *Assessing concepts of quality of care: results of a national survey of five self-regulating health professions in Canada*. CHEPA Working Paper Series No. 90–7, May, 1990, McMaster University, Hamilton, Ontario, Canada.
15. Hacon, W. S. The health manpower situation in Canada. Presented at the Pan American Conference on Health Manpower Planning, World Health Organization, Ottawa: September 10–14, 1973, p. 32.

16. Lalonde, M. A new perspective on the health of Canadians (White Paper). Ottawa, Government of Canada (April, 1974).
17. Hall, E. M. *Canada's national provincial health program for the 1980s: a commitment for renewal*. Ottawa, Supply and Services, 1980.
18. Adams, O. Present dilemma in manpower: the national perspective. Presented at the Medical Society of Prince Edward Island, 1988.
19. Anderson, G., Barer, M. and Kazanjian, A. Toward an integrated health human resource planning framework for Ontario. The University of British Columbia. Prepared for meeting of the expert panel to the Price Waterhouse Health Human Resources Planning Project.
20. Angus, D. E. An option for discussion: the Canadian health care system. Presented to the conference on who pays for a healthy America: health care options for the 1990s. Wichita, Kansas, 1990.
21. Angus, D. E. Review of significant health care commissions and task forces in Canada since 1983–84. Canadian Medical Association, Canadian Nursing Association and Canadian Hospital Association, Ottawa, 1990.
22. Barer, M. and Stoddart, G. Toward integrated medical resource policies for Canada. Report prepared for the Federal/Provincial/Territorial Conference of Deputy Ministers of Health. June, 1991, Canada.

CHAPTER 7

The cost savings–quality trade-off: empirical evidence of a cost–quality trade-off in the provision of community-based long-term care

Paul N. Rappoport[a] and
Arthur E. King[b]
[a]*Temple University, Philadelphia, and*
[b]*Lehigh University, Bethlehem, Pennsylvania, USA*

INTRODUCTION

In the USA the provision of community-based residential services for mentally retarded or developmentally disabled individuals represents a relatively recent model of long term care.[1] Prior to 1968 the mentally retarded were cared for at home or placed in state institutions with a primarily custodial level of service. Through a series of court decisions on the adequacy and quality of care, a number of states agreed to de-institutionalise and to embrace the concept of normalisation—placing clients in appropriate community-based residential

North American Health Care Policy in the 1990s
Edited by A. King, T. Hyclak, S. McMahon and R. Thornton

settings. The providers of these residential services were for the most part non-profit organisations with limited resources and experience in providing long-term care services. These providers were regulated and funded by state departments of mental retardation.

Through the 1970s and 1980s the demand for residential placement increased, as courts continued to follow more aggressive policies towards de-institutionalisation and access to services, following the actions brought forth by client advocates.[2] The costs of providing services increased faster than the funding. In an effort to deal with rapidly rising demand and the resulting costs, additional requirements were imposed on providers. Some of these requirements dramatically changed the way services were provided. For example, federally funded programmes for intermediate care facilities for the mentally retarded (ICF/MR) mandated that clients receive 'active programming' to ensure that clients were afforded the opportunity to develop to their potential level of functioning. For the first time, quality of care was highlighted as a necessary requirement for state and federal funding.

In the 1990s, this model was adapted to the realities of rising costs. Funding long-term care services for the developmentally disabled, previously 'mentally retarded', now was linked to cost containment, to tightened eligibility requirements, and, perhaps most importantly, to evidence of quality. Current policy represents at best a fragmented approach for dealing with potential trade-offs between quality and cost savings in the provision of long-term health care. On the one hand, some policies deal with cost control and, on the other, quality-assurance programmes are promoted quite independently of cost considerations as if no relationship exists between quality and cost savings. Further, focusing on a unified national health care policy may divert attention and funding away from some sub-sectors within the health care arena. This may well be the case for long-term care in general and specifically for care of the developmentally disabled. Thus, in the name of 'health care reform', policy-makers may actually diminish the quality of long-term care delivered.

Quality is a complex attribute that is intricately tied to the current debate on health care reform. Often, specific health care reforms are promoted or criticised because of their impact on the quality of delivered services, but without precisely defining quality or its behavioural relationship to the proposed reforms.[3] In this chapter, we seek to provide a conceptual model for the inclusion of quality and to apply it to the delivery of long-term care. Our objective is to provide support for the existence and extent of a quality–cost savings trade-off.

The next section describes the focus of this chapter, the regulatory background which provided the basis for the current market structure for long-term care and some of the relevant literature we draw upon for our model. We then develop the model from a theoretical perspective and show its transformation to an estimable form. The final section includes a discussion of the estimated results and some additional simulations with the model. In light of the empirical results, we discuss the interplay between quality and cost savings, and the implications for health care policy in the long-term care sector.

THE SETTING

Empirical Focus of this Study

Our analysis involves the evaluation of providers that offer residential services to the developmentally disabled who are funded through a state mental retardation programme, in this case, the Pennsylvania Office of Mental Retardation. Thus we do not focus on care purchased through the private network of providers. We selected the public segment of this health care market because: (i) the market for public long-term care is developing rapidly with the ageing population and rising cost of private care; (ii) providers who operate in this market are relatively homogeneous with respect to their size and services offered; (iii) budgeting is based primarily on a per diem or per client amount, thus enabling the direct computation of costs of service; (iv) service delivery and compliance are more easily monitored and measured; and, (v) this market appears to be targeted by the Health Care Financing Administration (HCFA) for a new level of service accountability in the near future.[4]

We focus on Pennsylvania for three reasons. First, one of the earliest original court cases involved the de-institutionalisation of clients at Pennhurst State Hospital (Philadelphia, PA). Consequently, Pennsylvania has one of the longest histories of community-based care for people with developmental disabilities. Second, the activism associated with de-institutionalisation led to the growth in firms providing residential services and the tracking of their experience under widely fluctuating levels of state and federal funding. Finally, there has been systematic data collection on programmes, clients and costs for over a decade in Pennsylvania, i.e. sufficient data were available for econometric analyses.

Previous Studies on Long-term Care

Studies of quality in long-term care settings have primarily focused on nursing homes and on community-based residential mental health programmes.[5] Kane and Kane noted that 'quality assurance in these long term care settings diverges from approaches used in acute care settings because of inherent features of long term care: slower pace, reliance on low technology services, and different goals of long term care.'[6] That is, the production function is different for long-term care and has fewer options for substitution among capital and labour than acute care. Generally a fixed-proportion functional form probably best describes the delivery of long-term health care services. In their study of quality-adjusted cost functions for nursing homes, Gertler and Waldman confirmed the very limited substitutability between capital and labour for their sample of 279 nursing homes in New York.[7]

Liu and McBridge, found in their study on the cost of

community care for disabled elderly persons that stringent eligibility requirements are critical for controlling costs.[8] Their study estimated the trade-off between specific activities of daily living deficiencies and cost. From the objective of minimising cost, they concluded that a national plan for long-term health care for this population would require cost controls as well as precise eligibility criteria. This study emphasises the costs associated with skilled nursing care, therapy and specialised services relative to personal and housekeeping care. Skilled care is expected to account for over 45% of the total cost per community care day.[9] Implicitly included is a cost–quality trade-off, seen through the substitution of less skilled for skilled services, in order to decrease the use of higher paid specialists. The very nature of the disabilities associated with this population, however, makes it unlikely that such substitutions are possible or even appropriate. As further evidence of limited substitutability, the share of programme budget associated with community-based facilities for the mentally retarded for direct care staff often exceeds 70%.[10]

Kane's characterisation of the differences between long-term care and acute-care settings[11] is applicable to an examination of the long-term care setting for the developmentally disabled (DD). In this setting, no specific acute-care episode exists and consequently no parallel measure to the set of 'outcomes' that measure quality of service for acute-care providers. The type of services required are determined primarily by the client's level of functioning. For lower-functioning clients, the services are close to custodial. For higher-functioning clients, the type of services available encompass vocational training and rehabilitation, and social rehabilitation. This segmentation by level of functioning is important in studying the provision of services to this population because the recent focus on quality in community settings has led to the evaluation of 'quality' based on the distinction between active treatment and passive, custodial treatment. Consequently, from an operational standpoint, the identification of appropriate outcomes is dependent on the level of functioning of the client.

The Regulatory Impetus for Community-based Care

Over the last two decades, community-based services have emerged as an alternative to institutional care.[12] Through consent decrees and federal legislation, states have been required to spend sizeable portions of their formula grants on deinstitutionalisation. A number of significant court cases including Willowbrook, Pennhurst, Pennsylvania Association for Retarded Citizens (PARC)[13] led the way for a series of consent decrees with numerous states which reinforced the place of community-based services in the provider marketplace. As attention focused on developmental disabilities through court initiatives, activity at the federal level increased with the passage of legislation for funding developmental disability programmes. The resulting legislation included the 1970 Developmental Disabilities Act, the 1973 Rehabilitation Act, the 1975 Developmental Disabilities Assistance Act, the 1978 Rehabilitation Act, Comprehensive Services and Developmental Disabilities Amendments, the 1984 Developmental Disabilities Act and the 1991 Handicapped and Disabilities Act.

In these celebrated cases, the courts accepted the principle of normalisation and applied it to the field of developmental disability. The principle of normalisation essentially dictated that the residential, educational and social conditions of an individual must be as close to the cultural norm for persons with a similar demographic profile as is reasonably possible—given a person's disability. The principle of normalisation was operationalised through the related concept of least restrictive alternative. This concept implied that developmentally appropriate care, training and support should be based on an individual's needs and to the maximum extent possible be provided in the types of community settings that are used by non-handicapped persons. The principle of least restrictive alternative was used successfully to argue for the deinstitutionalisation of both mentally ill and developmentally disadvantaged citizens.

The premise underlying all judicial efforts for de-institutionalisation and the fostering of the principle of least restrictive environment was the belief that community-based care is significantly better than institutional care. The reaction of the courts to the poor conditions found in state institutions led to their determination that quality of care could be increased by placing these individuals in community-based settings. De-institutionalisation was accepted and, in the process, created the provider market for community-based services met the new demand.

Noteworthy in the assessment of long-term care for the developmentally disabled was the active intervention of 'advocates' on behalf of the developmentally disabled. This intervention worked through the courts and resulted in pressures to expand the role of quality assurance as it applied to this constituency. Judicial advocacy resulted in services being mandated without regard to cost.[14]

Funding and Quality Assurance for Community-based Programmes

As this new industry developed, community-based housing and care were provided to those formerly in institutions. The providers were typically small, run by boards where there was at best limited business expertise, and where the organisations were typically underfunded. A majority of these providers had strong religious affiliations. A large segment of providers received nearly 100% of their funding from federal and state sources. The initial approach for funding these programmes was based on actual patient expenditures reimbursed on a per diem basis. This straightforward financing formula, while initially very appealing to these new service providers, later became burdensome as state agencies sought to curtail expenditures by restricting budgets. In particular, there were only limited provisions for modifying reimbursements for cost changes during the funding period, especially for overhead items such as insurance, transportation, debt service and rent.

From a policy standpoint, these community-based programmes owe their existence to judicial advocacy on the one hand and government funding on the other. There have been few problems with excess capacity in the industry because of the excess demand for placement as measured by the long waiting lists of eligible clients. A recent study by Beauregard and Potter verified the possibility of excess demand continuing into the late 1980s.[15] In 1987 while all community-based facilities had an occupancy rate of about 90%, group homes had a rate of 93%. In addition, an indirect measure of demand spillover effects was the fact that 16.7% of nursing home residents were diagnosed as mentally retarded and 24% of those were under age 55.[16] Thus the total number of patients in a state's facilities could be directly controlled by fiscal regulation of cost, budgets and eligibility criteria.

However, the overall costs of providing services increased rapidly because of the rapid growth of community placements, the reimbursement structure and the inexperience of government agencies in administering community-based programmes. This marketplace developed in the absence of accepted standards of quality of care and in the absence of adequate financial controls. Each state was left to budget and manage this market as best it could. The creation of ICF/MR programmes in 1971 as Title XIX of the Social Security Act marked shifts both in federal funding responsibility and in accountability with respect to operation of community programmes. This legislation quickly became the largest source of funding for community-based programmes.

With costs increasing states were forced to look for alternative funding sources and strategies for introducing cost savings. Converting community living arrangement facilities to Medicare-funded ICF/MR facilities enabled states to shift part of the cost of service to the federal government. Accompanying both the concern for cost containment and this shift in funding source was an increased requirement placed on providers of service to initiate quality-assurance (QA) programmes.

Initially, these QA programmes were designed to improve regulatory compliance. Approved organisational structure was viewed as the primary vehicle for assuring that minimal standards were met. For example, ICF/MR regulations required site visits and reviews as part of the licensing process. To monitor overall compliance, site reviewers were charged with the responsibility to determine: (i) the status of the residential facility; (ii) that health and safety rules and procedures were met; (iii) that documents were complete and organised; (iv) that the programme plan encouraged growth and development. This last component was designed to foster active treatment and client progress where possible even though standards for 'active treatment' had not been established. This criterion of active treatment and its lack of definition quickly became a controversial issue among the developmental disabilities specialists. In effect the Health Care Financing Administration (HCFA) was given the power to revoke licences of community-based providers if it was determined that care was only custodial or passive.

Long-term Care Programmes in Pennsylvania

Within Pennsylvania there are over 100 providers of residential and non-residential services to the developmentally disabled.[17] Of the 100 000–150 000 persons who need service, 45 000 mentally retarded persons receive them and over 15 000 have been placed in residential programmes. A majority of available services have been allocated to those who were de-institutionalised. For example, in fiscal 1988 over $400 million were allocated for community-based services.

In the absence of a definition for quality, Pennsylvania counties created task forces to operationalise quality assurance. Consider, for example, the definition of quality as developed by the Lehigh County (PA) mental retardation programme.[18] For managers of a mental retardation programme quality was defined to include:

1. Normalisation and client satisfaction.
2. Client participation in planning.

3. The delivery and monitoring of services.
4. The provision of health and safety services.
5. Client progress.

The general objectives that have been developed to frame quality were designed as open-ended:

1. Assuring that providers of service have the capability to provide acceptable levels of service.
2. Assuring that services are provided to clients in a manner which is consistent with good practice.
3. Assuring that the services that are provided have the intended affect.
4. Assuring that the legal and human rights of clients are protected.

It is within this background of advocacy, regulation and funding streams that our analysis of the cost savings–quality trade-off is cast. The model which we propose in the following section draws its structure from the institutional characteristics we have discussed.

A MODEL OF ENDOGENOUS QUALITY FOR LONG-TERM HEALTH CARE

Taxonomy of Quality

We begin in a similar fashion to Gertler and Waldman[19] (GW): they included quality as an explicit endogenous, but unobservable, variable in the cost function of a nursing home.[20] They noted that quality had been ignored in most analyses previously because of measurement and data availability problems.[21] In their conceptual model, they defined quality as one of two output attributes, the other being quantity. We agree with GW but argue that inclusion of one aggregate for quality is too limited a view of the perceptions of quality. The 'number of quality characteristics' is indeed large and complex, and is complicated by differing viewpoints from which quality attributes are perceived.

We propose a model which allows 'quality' to be subdivided by different groups of participating economic actors who derive utility from the provision of health care services. While we model long-term health care because it has a simpler fixed-proportions production structure than does acute care, we believe the model or an extension of it is applicable to acute care as well. GW were able to identify their empirical model with exogenous demand-shifting demographic variables for nursing homes[22] which were not available for our group of residential agencies for community-based care. Thus we take a different approach of specifying a structural behavioural model for utility maximisation by the publicly funded care-giving agency and then derive an estimable reduced form based on proxy variables.

Consider quality as perceived by four groups which derive utility from quality in the provision of health care:

Let: Q1 = client/patient-perceived quality of output of health care

This would be the closest type of quality to the traditional consumer-based, marketing-oriented concept originating from purchased product attributes. Also, it is closest to and most consistent with the traditional medical model where the patient 'gets well' more quickly, more happily and with higher-quality care.

Let: Q2 = labour/producer-perceived quality of health care as an input in the production process

Q2 depends on human capital factors such as quality and quantity of on-the-job training, job satisfaction, altruism of workers, etc.

Let: Q3 = organisation/firm/Agency[23]-perceived quality of health care services, including organising, administering and funding those services[24]

Q3 depends on Agency growth, survivability, reputation, altruism of administrators, etc. We explicitly recognise that the above three types of quality exist in a simultaneous, interdependent framework within the production process and the constraints of the funding process. GW implicitly use only the output interpretation of quality, similar to Q1 above, in their equation for output demand and in the derived cost function. Thus we can specify that:

Q3 = f(Q1, Q2, budget) = a composite view which includes binding constraints of financial and physical resources.

Finally, let:

Q4 = society's perceptions of quality of health care which include an understanding of the interdependence and trade-offs among system-wide objectives such as accessibility and affordability

If Agencies which comprise both providers and labour are to exist in the delivery system, they must be viable, which in turn requires both availability of financial resources and accounting flexibility. Furthermore, given the small scale of operation of many community-based Agencies or programmes relative to

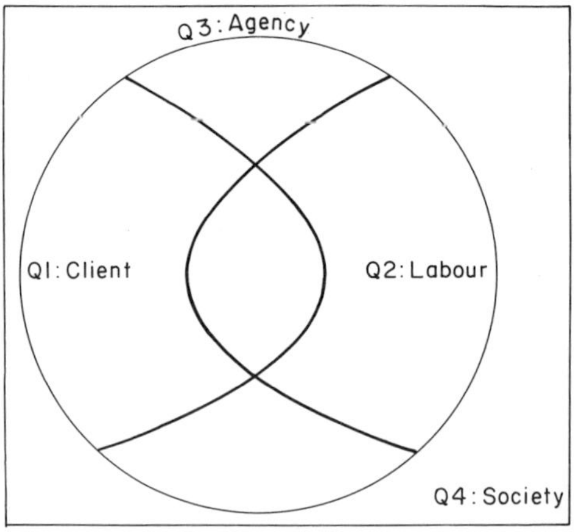

Figure 7.1 The taxonomy of quality

the entire delivery system, the regulation should not overburden the Agency manager(s).

For public policy makers to achieve society's goals and desired level of Q4, Q3 matters more than Q1 or Q2 separately. The interrelationship among all four types of quality is illustrated in Figure 7.1. Once society reaches some agreement on a social contract for an acceptable level of Q4, various policies can be implemented at the Agency level and the quality controlled through review, evaluation and other standard management techniques. Society controls Q4 and Q3 directly, but Q1 and Q2 indirectly through rules and regulations governing Q3.

A Model of Agency Utility Maximisation

Given:

$$Q1 = \text{client quality of output} = f(\text{CWB})$$

where CWB = client well-being;

$$Q2 = \text{staff quality of input} = f(\text{SS, CWB}, Z)$$

where SS = staff satisfaction, and Z = other job-related exogenous variables;

$$Q3 = \text{Agency quality} = f(\text{Q1, Q2, BC})$$

where BC = budget constraint.

Let:

$$\text{Agency utility} = \text{AU} = f(\#\text{clients}, \#\text{staff}, \text{Q1}, \text{Q2}, \text{Q3}) \quad (1)$$

where the function is non-additive;

$$\text{BC} = f(r \times \#\text{clients}, W \times \#\text{staff}) \quad (2)$$

where r = per capita reimbursement, and W = wage rate of staff.

However, given that the technology of long-term care is basically a fixed-factor, fixed-input–output ratio production process, and the funding process encourages full-capacity usage of the number of beds:

$$\#\text{staff} = f(F)$$

where F = number of clients. Then, with appropriate substitutions, the optimisation becomes:

$$\text{maximise AU} = f(\text{F, SS, Q1, Q2, Q3})$$

subject to $\text{BC} = f(r, W, F)$.

From the maximisation of Agency utility, there are three derived 'quality functions':

$$\text{Q1} = f(\text{SS}, F, \text{BC}, \text{CWB}) \tag{3}$$

$$\text{Q2} = f(W, \text{BC}, \text{SS}, \text{CWB}, Z) \tag{4}$$

$$\text{Q3} = f(\text{SS}, F, \text{BC}, Z) \tag{5}$$

Given that each quality dependent variable is highly correlated with one of its independent variables, we normalise these three quality functions:

$$\text{Q1}^* = g(\text{Q1}, \text{CWB}) = f(\text{SS}, F, \text{BC}) \tag{6}$$

$$\text{Q2}^* = h(\text{Q2}, \text{SS}) = f(\text{W}, \text{BC}, \text{CWB}, Z) \tag{7}$$

$$\text{Q3}^* = k(\text{Q3}, \text{BC}) = f(\text{SS}, F, Z) \tag{8}$$

In order to operationalise equations (6)–(8), we proxy quality by specific measures which are discussed in the next section:

$$g(\text{Q1}, \text{CWB}) = I = \text{measure of client progress}$$

$$h(\text{Q2}, \text{SS}) = S = \text{measure of staff involvement}$$

$$k(\text{Q3}, \text{BC}) = B = \text{measure of fiscal tightness}$$

We replace SS with S, and BC with B, as well. Thus, the no charge model becomes:

$$I = f(S, F, B) \tag{9}$$

$$S = f(W, B, I, Z) \tag{10}$$

$$B = f(S, F, Z) \tag{11}$$

Empirical Measures and Data

The view of quality that emerges from the above institutional and analytical discussions suggests that outcomes, process and structure are interdependent. The variables in equations (9)–(11) are specific to a facility or programme and thus require disaggregated client or staff-specific measures. We obtained data on 50 programmes in southeastern Pennsylvania and their 265 clients for the 1989–90 fiscal year. These programmes were group homes classified as either ICF/MRs or CLAs (community living arrangements) with an average size of five to six clients.

The measure for client well-being, *I*, was constructed from both information available on client intake forms and tests of client capabilities. Clients' information collected included demographics such as age, sex and extent of disabilities; level of functioning; previous placement history; medication history and other behavioural or maladaptive indicators. Outcome-based test scores were modified using a hedonic regression where hedonic modifiers included age, sex, previous history of institutionalisation and level of functioning.[25] The adjusted scores were organised by programme and averaged.

Staff involvement was proxied by the turnover rate, *S*. This choice was based on an extensive set of staff surveys which provided background information on staff attitudes and issues of concern to staff.[26] Additional staff demographics were also collected, including training, education level and previous experience. The relative wage rate, *W*, for direct care staff was computed as the ratio of the non-skilled service hourly wage rate to that of direct care staff. Related industries with alternative employment opportunities were fast food and retail establishments.[27] As is discussed further in the next section, supervisory longevity, *X*, was chosen as the job-related exogenous factor, specified as *Z* in equation (10). Both supervisory longevity, *X*, and overtime hours, OT, were specified as relating to the budget measure, *B*. As OT increases over the planned amount, it will become increasingly difficult for the programme manager(s) to meet the approved budget. Averages for *S*, *X* and OT were computed for each programme.

The programme-specific summary measure of budgetary performance, B, was computed from programme fiscal data. Accounting adjustments were made to ensure data comparability among all programmes. For example, programmes that were started in mid-year were pro-rated. Also, one-time, unexpected capital outlays, e.g. to repair wind storm damage, were also netted out. Budgetary performance was defined for programme-specific expenditures and did not include general overhead and administrative costs:

$$B = \frac{(\text{budgeted expenditures} - \text{actual expenditures})}{\text{budgeted expenditures}}$$

B greater than zero implies, purely from an accounting perspective, a fiscally well-managed programme. Size for our sample of programmes ranged from four to 16. The larger this measure, B, the more latitude Agency supervisors have in managing their programmes. However, if cost savings are required, say through reductions in the approved budgeted expenses, then B will decrease ($\partial B/\partial$ budget > 0). Furthermore, if the actual Agency spending increases beyond the budget, B declines ($\partial B/\partial$ actual expenses < 0).

The Operational Model and Testable Hypotheses

With the above measurements for each of the variables, our final, estimable model becomes:

$$I = f(S,\ F,\ B) \tag{12}$$

$$S = g(W,\ I,\ B,\ X) \tag{13}$$

$$B = h(S,\ F,\ X,\ \mathrm{OT}) \tag{14}$$

where I = hedonic index of client well-being; S = staff turnover; F = number of clients; B = measure of budgetary tightness; W = local services wage rate relative to direct-care wage rate; OT = overtime hours; and X = longevity of supervisor in years.

The testable hypotheses embodied in equation (12) imply that client well-being, once adjusted for demographics and level of functioning, depends on staff involvement (as measured by staff turnover), their residential/programme size, and the fiscal management of that programme. We expect $\partial I/\partial S < 0$, that higher turnover impedes client well-being. There is considerable anecdotal evidence that the stronger the binding and familiarity between clients and staff, the lower the turnover rate. Further, we hypothesise that smaller programmes are more easily managed, i.e. $\partial I/\partial F < 0$. Finally, the better fiscally managed the programme, the more discretion supervisors have, for example, to organise special enrichment activities or improve existing ones, and clients will benefit more. Thus we hypothesise that $\partial I/\partial B > 0$.

Equation (13) models staff turnover as a function of relative wage rates (W), management of the programme (B), client well-being (I) and supervisor longevity (X). We expect an inverse relationship between management of the facility and staff turnover, $\partial S/\partial B < 0$, because well-managed programmes would be less stressful to employees, requiring fewer sacrifices or changed behaviour, and thereby significantly lower the staff turnover rate. If the direct-care staff member has the opportunity to earn more in other service-related jobs, with higher relative wages, then $\partial S/\partial W > 0$, which follows standard labour market behaviour. Finally, we expect lower turnover rates in programmes with 'good' supervisors, $\partial S/\partial X < 0$, whom we presume are well organised, interpersonally skilled and engender confidence in their subordinates.

In equation (14) the management of a programme as measured by a programme's ability to stay on budget, B, is hypothesised to be a function of turnover (S), overtime hours (OT), the experience of the supervisor (X) and the size of the program (F). We expect a programme's fiscal performance to be positively related to the experience of the programme supervisor ($\partial B/\partial X > 0$), negatively related to overtime hours ($\partial B/\partial \mathrm{OT} < 0$) and negatively related to staff turnover ($\partial B/\partial S < 0$). The relationship of programme size (F) and budget management is unclear *a priori*. For example, if there are economies of scale, larger programmes would be more likely to have more flexibility to rearrange their budgets and thereby avoid unplanned deficits. On the other hand, larger programmes may have a more difficult case mix to manage, putting pressure on case workers and supervisory staff and leading in turn to costly decisions which could adversely affect budget allocations.

The resulting three-equation model of quality enables the direct testing of the linkages between client outcomes and staff turnover, and from staff turnover to programme budget management. From a health policy staff viewpoint, turnover and programme management are two variables which have practical implications for the implementation of specific policy changes. For example, turnover rates are readily measurable by funding and Agency officials. These rates can be segmented by size of programme, programme management and by length of service. They can be related to wage rates and alternative labour opportunities. Budgets can be likewise tracked and monitored. Second, these variables are at least partially under the control of the programme or Agency. High turnover rates provide direct evidence for bringing direct-care staff wage rates in line with competitive alternatives. Thus Agency budgets must be increased and the pressure for cost savings decreased. If the linkage of turnover to client well-being proves to be statistically significant, this would provide a strong and tangible argument for more funding for direct-care staff training and career development. Budget management is essential if a programme is to meet state-mandated levels of programme compliance. Early detection of a programme which is 'out of control' may be possible if the linkages back to staff turnover and client progress are statistically strong. Third, these measures are readily observable in daily operations and should be understandable to both staff and management, thereby facilitating implementation of programme improvements.

EMPIRICAL RESULTS

Two-stage Least-squares Estimates of Model Parameters

Our final three-equation model, (12)–(14), is an interdependent system with I, S and B jointly determined with exogenous variables W, X, O and F. Because the model is identified by the rank condition and over-identified by the order condition, two-stage least squares was used to estimate the parameters. Results are presented below.[28] The two-stage least-squares standard errors are reported below each estimate and the t-ratios at the bottom.

Client well-being (12)

$$
\begin{array}{lllllll}
I = & -\ 0.649 & -\ 0.153\,S & -\ 0.252\,F & +\ 0.249\,B & & R^2 = 0.79 \\
 & (1.700) & (0.049) & (0.121) & (0.053) & & F = 9.08 \\
 & -\ 0.382 & 3.142 & -\ 2.088 & 4.670 & &
\end{array}
$$

Staff turnover (13)

$$
\begin{array}{lllllll}
S = & 0.649 & -\ 0.645\,B & +\ 1.071\,W & -\ 0.099\,I & -\ 0.011\,X & R^2 = 0.69 \\
 & (0.036) & (0.054) & (0.070) & (0.029) & (0.002) & F = 67.45 \\
 & 18.122 & -\ 11.898 & 15.283 & -\ 3.386 & -\ 4.639 &
\end{array}
$$

Budgetary performance (14)

$$
\begin{array}{lllllll}
B = & -\ 1.091 & -\ 1.022\,S & -\ 0.865\,\mathrm{OT} & +\ 0.199\,X & +\ 0.501\,F & R^2 = 0.86 \\
 & (0.387) & (0.064) & (0.246) & (0.087) & (0.245) & F = 20.61 \\
 & -\ 2.817 & -\ 16.041 & -\ 3.511 & 2.293 & 2.048 &
\end{array}
$$

Discussion of Results: Individual Equations and Coefficients

In evaluating these estimated coefficients we first focused on the sign of the explanatory variable, then the statistical significance of the entire relationship embodied in each single equation using the t and F tests. On the basis of these tests all coefficients are significant at the 5% level and many are significant at better than the 1% level. Furthermore, the *a priori* reasoning about each coefficient sign discussed above is confirmed by the estimates. After some additional comments about the results of the individual equations, we present two simulations with this model to demonstrate the effects of the simultaneous interactions of the three endogenous variables.

Each equation in the model provides a means for assessing three interdependent dimensions of quality from the perspective of provider management. Equation (14) looks at the relationship, *ceteris paribus*, of budgets, programme size and staff stability on client well-being. Whereas from the programmatic perspective, client well-being depends on the client's programming and level of support and services, nonetheless we find Agency variables to be statistically important. That is, cut-backs in approved budgets, i.e. increased cost savings, or the inability to manage actual expenditures will lead to an overall decrease in client well-being, as measured by our hedonic index, I. This is an important result because we have demonstrated a strong statistically significant direct relationship between B, representing costs, and I: as cost savings decrease, B increases, thereby increasing quality of client well-being. This empirical evidence of a cost savings–quality trade-off should be a useful guide for health care policy-makers, especially with the estimate of its magnitude provided in the next section.

Programme size (F) represents a two-edged sword. In terms of client well-being, size has a negative impact—the larger the programme the lower the overall average client well-being. However, in terms of overall fiscal management, B, programme size is positive, indicating larger programmes have budgets which will more likely be managed and maintained. This may be from the fiscal perspective some evidence of scale economies in operation of a residential long-term care facility.

Staff turnover emerges as a key significant variable in the modelling of quality. An increase in staff instability, as measured by an increase in the turnover rate, decreases overall client well-being. Staff instability increases when relative wage rates from competing job opportunities rise. In addition, the inverse relationship to the overall fiscal management of the programme implies the importance to direct care staff and a successful programme of careful management of staff hours and the promotion of team-work.

Improved fiscal effectiveness, *B*, clearly depends on low staff turnover and the sparing use of overtime hours. As noted earlier, however, programme size partly offsets the overtime and staff turnover effects. Supervisory longevity, implying an ability to manage an overall programme, has a positive impact on fiscal effectiveness. Supervisory longevity helps moderate staff instability.

Policy Simulations with the Model

In order both to evaluate the model's robustness with respect to the estimation of an equation system representing quality and to assess the usefulness of the model for policy analyses, we have performed two realistic simulations with the estimated model. For the first policy scenario, we estimated the magnitude of the trade-off between cost savings and quality by simulating the effect of worsening the programme budgetary pressure, *B*, by 1%. In effect we increased unplanned expenditures without a corresponding increase in budget. Then in order to study the problem of labour market competition for direct-care workers, we simulated the overall effect of a 1% rise in the wage of alternative jobs relative to that of direct-care workers.

With *B* cut by 1%, the most important result shown in Figure 7.2 is that we have again demonstrated the existence of a trade-off between cost savings/budget pressure and quality/client well-being: *I* diminishes by 1.35%. The staff turnover is inversely related to the budget cut, with an elasticity of −5.54%. Thus, when funding is cut for long-term residential health care, clients suffer, workers exit to other jobs and managers must scramble to make short-term adjustments in remaining workers' schedules.[29]

When relative wages for unskilled workers increase, as has

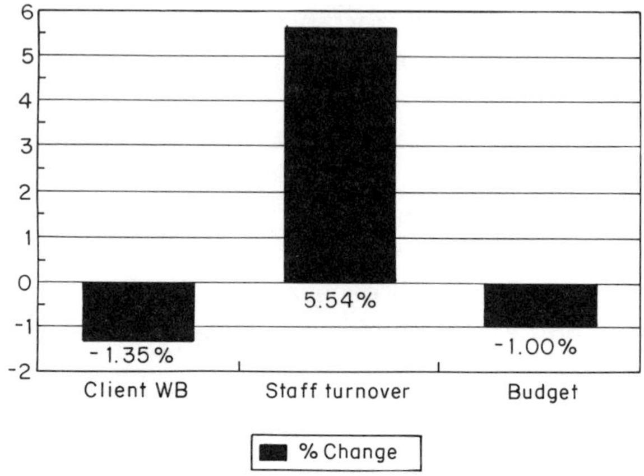

Figure 7.2 Budget reduction simulation: fiscal tightening scenario

been the case in recent years, the effect of this labour market shift is to increase staff turnover, decrease client well-being (quality of care) and put unplanned pressure on the programme's ability to stay within budget. The results for a 1% increase in *W* are illustrated in Figure 7.3. With the elasticity of staff turnover with respect to relative wages at almost 18%, the

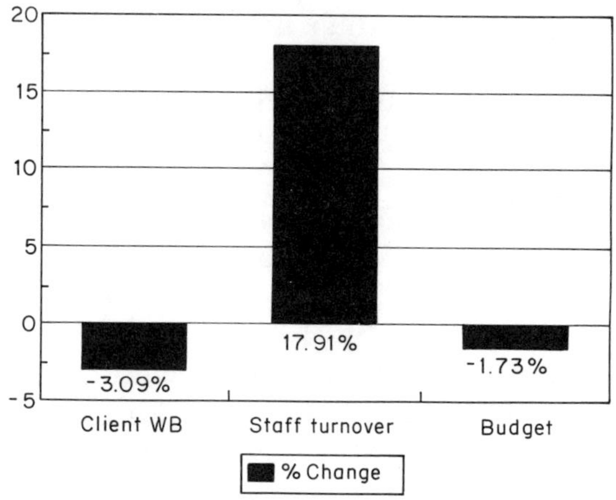

Figure 7.3 Relative wage simulation: decline in direct care staff relative wage

volatility of the labour market for direct-care workers is underscored. The strong cross-effects of labour instability were noted on client well-being, as *I* declines by 3%. The fiscal impact was less pronounced, but nonetheless adverse, as actual expenditures, e.g. for overtime, would have increased relative to approved budgets.

CONCLUSIONS

The identification of quality and its measurement is critical to the delivery of long-term care which is produced with a very high proportion of direct-care labour. Quality as a concept is open to multiple views, and many characterisations of quality are not easily made operational or even measurable. The model we have presented nonetheless provides a practical means for examining quality from the perspective of budgets and staffing. Quality as viewed from the perspective of our interdependent equation system suggests a number of practical implications. First, the model quantifies the importance of fiscal management. Quality appears to be highly dependent on budget funding and the effective use of those dollars. Whereas this finding is not necessarily surprising in general, the significance of the direct impact on client well-being should warn those who advocate active treatment that a cut in resources—increased cost savings—for such treatment will lead to diminished client progress. Those resources include nurses, physical therapists and other professionals experienced with the treatment of developmental disabilities.

Also, the role both direct-care staff and supervisory staff play in this environment is significant. Direct-care staff are classified as unskilled labour and are paid accordingly. Efforts have proceeded in a number of states to raise their relative wage rate. However, with states currently in the depth of their own fiscal crises, the ability of health policy-makers to respond has been limited. Even if they can stabilise direct-care staff turnover, there is no guarantee of improved quality. However, the evidence suggests that moderating turnover rates is an enabling condition for client progress. There is, then, a case which can be made on behalf of programme administrators that quality can be achieved and maintained but not when budgets are cut, or when direct-care staff wage rates are allowed to fall below comparable wage rates.

Whereas quality has many facets, this model provides direct evidence of a cost savings–quality trade-off: budgets matter, staff turnover matters, and wages matter. These trade-offs must be taken into account when programmes are created and administered. Furthermore, the size of such trade-offs must be considered by courts who favour de-institutionalisation and by programme advocates who wish to expand the opportunities for the disabled in order to promote reasonable levels of economic resources to achieve valued goals of providing quality health care.

ACKNOWLEDGEMENTS

The authors wish to acknowledge the following sources of assistance for the research on this chapter. This research was initiated during Rappoport's sabbatical from Temple University, Department of Economics, at the Community Foundation for Human Development (Sellersville, PA); appreciation is offered to Dr. David Austin, Executive Director of CFHD. King's financial support was provided by Lehigh University's Canadian Studies Program, the Martindale Center for the Study of Private Enterprise and the Department of Economics. Comments by John Hutton and Alan Maynard on earlier drafts of this chapter were appreciated. The authors absolve all of the above from any remaining difficulties in this chapter.

REFERENCES

1. See Kane, R. L., Lessons in long-term care: the benefits of a northern exposure. *Health Economics* 1992; **1(2)**: 105–114, for a description of the current Canadian situation.

2. For recent commentary on the advocacy-based approach, see Maynard, A., Health care reform in the United States, *Health Economics*, 1992, **1(3)**: 147–148.
3. For example, many practical discussions on quality assurance stress the delivery of reliable and appropriate services at a reasonable cost. Nowhere is 'reasonable' defined.
4. See Smith, D., Quality assurance: a review of historical trends in state and federal initiatives. Paper presented at the IBM conference on Quality Assurance: Concepts, Theory and Measurement, Harrisburg, PA, November, 1990. Also, see Health Care Financing Administration (June 3, 1988), *Medicaid Program Conditions for Intermediate Care Facilities for the Mentally Retarded: Final Rule*, Federal Register, **53(107)**: 20448–20505.
5. See, for example, Rothbard, A. B., Schinnar, A. P., Hadley, T. R. and Rovi, J., Integration of mental health data on hospital and community services, *Administration and Policy in Mental Health* 1990; **18(2)**: 91–99.
6. Kane, R. L. and Kane, R. A. Long-term care: variations on a quality assurance theme. *Inquiry* 1988; No. 25: 133.
7. Gertler, P. J. and Waldman, D. M. Quality adjusted cost functions, p. 11, NBER Working Paper No. 3567 (December, 1990). We discuss their model further in the text as a starting point for our own model.
8. Liu, K. and McBridge, T. Cost of community care for disabled elderly persons: the policy implications. *Inquiry* 1990; No. 27: 65.
9. Liu and McBridge, op. cit., pp. 67–68.
10. Theodore Poister Associates. *A Cost Function Analysis of Private Residential Services for Mentally Retarded Persons in the Commonwealth of Pennsylvania*, 1988.
11. Kane, R. L., op. cit., pp. 105–106.
12. See Castellani, P., *The Political Economy of Developmental Disabilities*, (Baltimore, Brooks, MD 1990) pp. 11–34, for documentation of the creation of this market.
13. Castellani, P., op. cit., p. 15.
14. For example, consideration of cost comparisons between community and institutional care was non-existent at this time. In 1986, anecdotal evidence from interviews with Canadian health economists suggested that politicians were still supporting community care on the basis of cost-cutting rather than improved quality. Kane, R. L., op. cit., p. 111, noted that '[i]f the full costs are considered [e.g. case management], community care is usually more expensive'.
15. Beauregard, K. and Potter, D. E. B. *Characteristics of Facilities for the Mentally Retarded*, AHCPR Publication No. 92-0067; National

Medical Expenditure Survey Data Summary 6, Agency for Health Care Policy and Research, Rockville, MD, (September, 1992) pp. 4–7.

16. Lair, T. *A Profile of Nursing Home Users Under Age 65*, AHCPR Publication No. 92-0060; National Medical Expenditure Survey Research Finding 13, Agency for Health Care Policy and Research, Rockville, MD (August, 1992) pp. 5–7.
17. See, for example, the membership directory of the Pennsylvania Association of Resources for People with Mental Retardation (PAR), Harrisburg, PA, 1990, for a summary of the scope of the mental retardation care provider market. See also *State Budget Requests 1988–89* and *Annual Report*, 1988–90, PA Office of Mental Retardation.
18. *The Lehigh County Mental Retardation Program Quality Assurance Plan of Action*, 1988. Similar views are expressed by the Human Services Research Institute, in *Assessing and Enhancing the Quality of Human Services*, 1984. Nowhere in these guides do the authors focus on direct-care workers or cost.
19. Gertler, P. J. and Waldman, D. M., op. cit., pp. 3–4, present a model in which quality appears initially in the demand function.
20. Braeutigam, R. and Pauly, M. Cost function estimation and quality bias: the regulated automobile industry. *Rand Journal of Economics* 1986; **17**: 606–617, provides one of the first analyses of a model with endogenous quality as an explicit argument.
21. They solve the problem of available data by defining quality as a latent (unobservable, i.e. not requiring data) variable and proceed to estimate the model based on a maximum likelihood estimator. Latent variable techniques are specifically designed to provide estimates without data on all endogenous variables. See Greene, W. H. *Econometric Analysis*, New York, Macmillan, 1990, pp. 531–537 for more information.
22. Gertler, P. J. and Waldman, D. M., op. cit., pp. 5–10.
23. We use 'Agency' as the firm producing the residential health care services, as is commonly used to describe the funded administrators. We do not wish to confuse it with *a*gency, which is the interpersonal relationship between a patient/client and the staff or administration.
24. We do not distinguish between Agency perceptions of quality and those of the funding source, although there may be disparities between these two groups.
25. See Goldman, F. and Grossman, M., The demand for pediatric care: an hedonic approach. *Journal of Political Economy* 1979; 259–261; and Hartman, R. and Doane, M., The use of hedonic analysis for certification and damage calculations in class action

complaints. *Journal of Law, Economics and Organization* 1987; **3(2)**: 360, for examples. Our outcome-based measure of client well-being reflected the programming and how the client responded to it, client progress and, to a lesser extent, client satisfaction. The hedonic index *I* is directly related to client well-being.

26. These surveys were made while Rappoport was associated with the Community Foundation for Human Development, Sellersville, PA. A brief synopsis of key findings which support our use of turnover as a measure of staff involvement is available from the authors. Additional survey work—with 674 clients, 245 direct-care staff and 44 supervisors—of factors which influence client well-being revealed statistically significant relationships with staff attitude and both staff and supervisor longevity. These factors attest to the importance of a stable labour-force when considering client well-being.
27. Data on the appropriate alternative jobs were available on exit surveys of leaving workers from the Community Foundation for Human Development.
28. The software package Soritec was used for the estimation. Note the reported $\bar{R}^2$ should be interpreted with care, because R^2 is not completely comparable to that computed for ordinary least squares unless the system is exactly identified. See Theil, H., *Principles of Econometrics*, New York, Wiley, 1971, for a further discussion.
29. Presumably, another round of simulation could show the effects of the predictable need to increase overtime hours (OT), an exogenous variable and not subject to induced changes in this model.

CHAPTER 8

Forces for reforming the US health care system: a review of the cost and access issues*

Susan M. Browning
American Medical Association, Chicago, Illinois, USA

INTRODUCTION

The American health care system has a long-standing reputation as one of the most advanced and sophisticated in the world. Patients seek state-of-the-art treatment from the nation's premier medical centres and specialists. Physicians and medical students from other countries are drawn to teaching hospitals and universities in the USA to learn the most advanced medical procedures and emerging technologies. And the overwhelming majority of Americans express strong satisfaction with the medical care provided by their family physicians.[1,2]

Despite these medical achievements, criticisms of the American health care system have grown over the past decade.

* The views expressed in this chapter are those of the author and may not represent those of the American Medical Association.

North American Health Care Policy in the 1990s
Edited by A. King, T. Hyclak, S. McMahon and R. Thornton

These criticisms have focused on two perceived deficiencies of the current system. First, total health spending commands an increasing share of the nation's resources despite numerous cost-containment measures implemented by payers throughout the 1980s. In 1989, health care consumed 11.6% of US gross national product (GNP),[3] a much higher proportion than other industrial countries devoted to health care.[4] Second, a growing number of Americans have limited financial access to health care; that is, they are uninsured and ineligible for public health programmes such as Medicaid. This uninsured population grew by 30% between 1978 and 1989.[5] Recent estimates place the number of Americans lacking private or public insurance at 33.4 million, or about 13.6% of the total population.[6]

These fundamental challenges of rising costs and declining access to care have led to many proposals for changing the current financing and delivery of health care in the USA. The goals, mechanisms and comprehensiveness of the reform ideas often vary substantially. Some proposals focus on improving access to care for the uninsured; others concentrate more on developing new incentives to control health care spending. Many of the proposals recommend incremental changes of the current pluralistic financing system through tax and regulatory policies and Medicaid expansion; others call for a fundamental restructuring of the system into a single or all-payer scheme. All of the proposals are being advanced and debated in the expectation that the USA will undertake some type of legislative health care reform initiative within the next several years.

This chapter reviews the two major forces driving the health care reform debate. The first section examines the cost issue and discusses trends in national health care expenditures, causes of rising health care costs, and the impact of rising expenditures on the major purchasers of health care, government and business. The second section examines the access issue and discusses sources of health insurance coverage, the demographic characteristics of the uninsured population, and the reasons why individuals lack health coverage. This review of the cost and access issues should facilitate an understanding of the perceived problems with the current health care system and the potential effects of alternative policy solutions offered by advocates in the American health care reform debate.

HEALTH CARE COSTS

Trends in Health Care Expenditures

In 1989, the USA spent $604.1 billion on health care. This amount was almost two and a half times the $249.1 billion spent in 1980.[7] Growth in health care spending also accelerated steadily throughout most of the 1980s. After adjusting for inflation, the annual real rate of growth in health care spending was 5.4% from 1980 to 1989.[8] In terms of 1989 dollars, real health care spending per capita rose from $950 in 1970 to $2,354 in 1989, an average annual rate of growth of about 4.9% .[5] By comparison, real rates of growth in other sectors of the economy have been much smaller during these same years (1970–1988). Spending for food increased at an average annual rate of about 1% , and spending for housing increased at an average annual rate of 3%.[9]

National health care expenditures have also risen faster than most other components of the economy. As a result, health spending commands an increasing share of GNP, from 9.1% of GNP in 1980 to 11.6% in 1989.[3,9] Further, although the service sector, in general, expanded as a share of GNP throughout the 1980s, health care services increased at twice the rate of all other services.[8] Government officials estimate that health spending will reach 15% of GNP by the year 2000 in the absence of any significant change in current trends.[9]

International comparisons[10]

Most other industrial nations spend less on health care than the USA. In 1989, US per capita spending on health care was $2354; 40% higher than Canada ($1683), 91% higher than Germany ($1232), and 182% higher than that spent in the UK

($836).[4] Similarly, the share of national output devoted to health care is substantially higher in the USA than in these other industrial countries. In 1989, the USA spent 11.8% of its gross domestic product (GDP)[11] on health care. In that same year, the proportion of GDP devoted to health care was 8.7% in Canada, 8.2% in Germany, and 5.8% in the UK.[4]

Despite the higher levels of spending, gross measures of health status are not comparatively better in the USA. Life expectancy in the USA is about the same or slightly shorter than in many other developed countries, including Canada, France, Germany, Japan and the UK. The USA infant mortality rate also compares unfavourably to other industrial nations; among 22 countries in the Organisation for Economic Cooperation and Development for whom infant mortality data are reported, the US ranks 15th.[12]

These international comparisons have prompted some questions about the effectiveness of the American health care system and the value of the nation's higher per capita spending. Life expectancy and infant mortality statistics, however, are influenced by many factors beyond access to and receipt of health care—including income, occupation, education, genetics, behavioural patterns and lifestyle trends. Therefore, the relatively less favourable US rates may reflect more about social issues and lifestyle characteristics than about the effectiveness of the health care provided.[13]

Causes of Rising Health Care Expenditures

The growth in health care spending in the USA has been influenced by such factors as medical care price inflation, widespread health insurance coverage, new technologies, 'defensive medicine', and the overall growth and ageing of the population. Some factors, such as economic and demographic changes, are external to the health care system and therefore not easily changed by health policy. Other factors, however, are internal to the health care sector and play a key role in some of the proposed reform strategies to control national expenditure and utilisation growth. As background for understanding the issues, all of the factors are reviewed below, with a discussion of some of the underlying forces that influence them.

Medical care price inflation

Medical prices in the USA have risen consistently faster than the prices of other goods and services in the economy. As measured by the Consumer Price Index (CPI), prices for medical care increased 66% more than prices for all consumer items between 1965 and 1989. From 1980 to 1989, the CPI for medical care increased by 99% compared to 46% for shelter, 33% for transportation, and 40% for food.[14]

These relative price increases often are a 'red flag' in discussions of national health spending. There are, however, two explanations for the relatively rapid increase in medical care prices. First, wages in the health care sector have risen faster than in the rest of the economy. While wages in most industries failed to keep pace with inflation during the 1980s, rank-and-file health care workers (16 years of schooling or less) did comparatively better, surpassing employees in the rest of the economy by 1.3% per year from 1979 to 1985.[15] Second, the health care sector is primarily a service industry characterised by lower productivity growth than manufacturing industries—a phenomenon attributed to the labour intensity of service production. Manufacturing industries have realised productivity gains over the past century, largely from the routinisation of production and the substitution of capital for labour. This productivity growth helps offset wage increases and tends to keep the prices of commodities low relative to the prices of services. In the health care sector, however, productivity growth has been relatively slower, thus contributing to medical care price inflation above the rate of inflation in the overall economy.[16]

Perhaps more importantly, the relative increase in the price of medical care reflects improvements in the quality of services over time. However, the CPI Medical Care Market Basket does not adjust for all such quality changes nor does it measure the exact same product over time. As Joseph Newhouse recently stated:

> From artificial hips, to noninvasive diagnostic machines, to improved mortality rates for childhood leukemias, to TPA [tissue plasminogen activator] for heart attacks, we are not pricing a product whose characteristics do not change. Because a correction is rarely made for these improvements, part of what we term a price increase is instead improved quality. How much the improved quality is worth it is a difficult issue, but the current index usually pretends it is not worth anything and that the additional expenditure is pure inflation.[17]

Therefore, the failure to account for quality improvements may bias medical care price inflation upward, relative to economy-wide inflation. Although the CPI for all items suffers from the same bias, the rapid increases in technology and services in the health care sector make it less likely that quality improvements will be captured in the CPI for medical care.

Health insurance

The spread of private health insurance, especially during the 1950s and 1960s, has been a major factor in rising health care expenditures in the USA. Health insurance reduces the price of care to patients and encourages them to consume more care than they would without coverage.[18,19] From 1950 to 1970, the proportion of hospital expenses paid out-of-pocket by patients dropped by 30%.[20] By 1987, patients' share of each dollar devoted to hospital care was, on average, about 10 cents; their share of dollars paid to physicians was about 26 cents.[19] The decreased price responsiveness (e.g. lower out-of-pocket expenses for medical care) and the increased demand for care in the presence of insurance coverage also drives up the price of medical care. These higher prices create greater incentives for more comprehensive health insurance to protect individuals from incurring substantial health care expenses at time of illness.[5]

The current tax treatment of employer-sponsored health insurance, which exacerbates individual incentives to 'over-consume' health care, has also influenced the growth in health care spending. Employer-sponsored health benefits are a non-taxable benefit to employees (and a tax-deductible business expense for firms). This tax treatment of non-cash compensation is effectively an employee subsidy for the purchase of insurance coverage that encourages individuals to obtain more generous insurance coverage than they would otherwise purchase, given a cash equivalent amount and their expected medical needs.[21] The richer benefit packages, in turn, provide additional incentives for the privately insured to consume more health care services.

The net effect of insurance on demand and health care use, however, varies widely depending on the individual's scope of covered services, plan deductibles, co-payments, and other limits on patient financial liability. Further, while the expansion of insurance has significantly increased the likelihood of seeking medical care, research has shown that the effect on expenditures per episode of care has been much smaller.[20] Therefore, while private and public insurance programmes have undoubtedly contributed to the rise in national health spending, there is some uncertainty about the direct effect and relative magnitude of insurance on expenditure growth.

Technology

Advance in technology has been an important factor in rising health care expenditures. New diagnostic equipment and therapeutic interventions have been rapidly introduced and widely disseminated in the health care sector during the last three decades. Some of these advances reflect a new 'product' in health care and permit formerly impossible interventions. Other innovations improve on existing diagnostic and medical therapies or reduce the pain or risk of certain invasive procedures. In general, new technology, while providing benefit to patients, increases the number of potential candidates for therapy and adds to the average and total costs of care.[19] For example, the cost of AZT, a drug which can delay the onset of AIDS in patients who test positive for human immunodeficiency virus, is estimated to be about $5 billion annually.[22]

Other experts, however, caution against the blanket endorsement of emerging technology as 'cost-enhancing'.[23] Some advancements which substitute non-invasive procedures for complicated surgical techniques have brought a clear reduction in treatment prices for selected medical conditions. The introduction of antibiotics, for example (perhaps one of the leading innovations of the twentieth century), decreased medical treatment costs and increased survival rates for many common diseases. But the general consensus is that technological innovation contributes to rising health care expenditures by expanding the number of beneficial interventions available and by decreasing the invasiveness of existing procedures—thus increasing the *number* of potential patients who stand to benefit from diagnosis or treatment.

Demographic influences

The total US population has been growing at about 1% per year, leading to a natural, albeit small, increase in health care expenditures. More importantly, the proportion of the population over 65 has grown consistently. Typically, the elderly have greater health care needs than the young and generate much higher average health care expenses. In 1987, for example, per capita health care spending was $745 for people under age 19, compared with $5360 for those age 65 and over and $9178 for people age 85 or over.[24] And expenditures are particularly high very late in life: about 30% of total Medicare expenditures are spent on the 6% of enrollees who are in their last year of life.[25] Because health care consumption rises sharply with age, the increase in the proportion of the population over age 65 has pushed up USA national health spending. This demographic trend is expected to continue into the next century and will most likely lead to further expenditure growth.

Malpractice premiums, 'defensive medicine' and consumer demand

Professional liability insurance premiums have grown at an annual rate of about 15% in recent years, totalling $5.1 billion in 1989.[26] These increases in provider costs, which are often indirectly passed on to patients, have undoubtedly contributed to some of the growth in national health spending.

More important to total spending, however, is the practice of 'defensive medicine' by providers to protect themselves from possible malpractice claims. The American Medical Association estimated that the costs of defensive medicine activities (including more extensive record keeping, spending more time with patients, and ordering additional tests or services) totalled $15.1 billion in 1989. Together, malpractice premiums and defensive medicine were $20.2 billion, or about 18% of all physician service expenditures in that year.[26] The malpractice environment, therefore, has boosted total health care spending beyond what would have been expected in the absence of the current system of adversary litigation.

Consumer demand for health care has also influenced the volume of services and expenditures per capita. Consumers have become increasingly sophisticated about health care, raising their expectations of and desire for high quality, 'high tech' services. Widespread media dissemination of information on the advances in health care and the availability of new treatments in local communities continue to foster consumer awareness and influence the demand for health care services.

The 'Burden' of Rising Health Care Outlays

Trends in US health care expenditures and the continued escalation of medical care prices have been a source of widespread concern among the major purchasers of health care, government and business. Although their share of total health carespending has been fairly stable throughout the 1980s, other indicators show that health care costs have become a more significant expense, or 'burden', for these payers.

The government perspective

Government is the largest third-party payer of health care. In 1989, federal, state and local governments paid $253.3 billion for health care, funding about 41.9% of the nation's health care bill.[28] Increases in government revenue, however, have not kept pace with increases in government health spending over the past decades. Government spent 5% of its general revenue on health care in 1965; by 1989, this share had increased to 14.8%.[3]

Health expenditures also represent a growing share of the federal budget. Compared with other major components of the domestic budget, the share devoted to health care increased at a rate second only to interest on the national debt during the 1980s.[8] Federal outlays for health accounted for 7.6% of the total federal budget in 1970; by 1990, this percentage had risen to 13.4%.[29] Increased Medicare expenditures during the 20-year period accounted for much of this growth. In 1990, the Medicare programme represented 7.8% of total federal budget outlays and almost 60% of all health outlays.

These indicators have fuelled public sector interest in reform of the nation's health care system. Growing concern about a relatively fixed public budget in the near term, based on the size of the federal debt and the near-universal voter opposition to tax increases, further contributes to the perceived need for reform. Many reform advocates also contend that as the USA directs more resources into the production of health care, investment in other areas that compete for public dollars, including education, housing, and transportation, will be compromised.[30]

The employer perspective

In 1989, employers spent $176.8 billion on health care benefits for workers, retirees, and their dependents, accounting for 29.3% of total national health care spending.[31] Health care benefits are currently the fastest-growing component of employee compensation. And employer health expenditures as a percentage of wages and salaries more than tripled from 1965 to 1989, from 2.2% to 8.3%.[3]

Additionally, concerns over the effect of growing health benefit costs on American competitiveness have prompted business's interest in restructuring the current health care system. Many corporations contend that rising health costs translate into relatively higher prices for American products, undermining international competitiveness. Chrysler Corporation, for example, reports that health insurance benefits (for Chrysler workers and Chrysler parts makers) accounted for $700 of the price of every new car produced in 1987. Reported estimates for health costs of foreign producers were substantially lower in that same year: $375 per car in France, $337 in Germany, and $246 in Japan.[29]

Some economists, however, argue that health care costs should not be singled out any more than wages—a much larger part of total employee compensation—in terms of their effect on product price and international competition.[32] Following this argument, fringe benefits and cash compensation are viewed as substitutes for one another in a well-functioning market; thus increases in health benefit costs can be passed on to employees in the long run. Douglas Fraser, past president of the United Auto Workers Union, summarised this argument in a recent health policy debate:

> Before you start weeping for the auto companies and all they pay for medical insurance, let me tell you how the system works. All company bargainers worth their salt keep their eye on the total labour unit cost ... [what they pay for health care] is money that can't be spent for higher [cash] wages or higher pensions or other fringe benefits.[33]

The economic perspective and the efficiency arguments

As noted, the health care sector's share of GNP rose from 5.9% in 1965 to 11.6% in 1989.[3,9] There is widespread belief that some of this growth reflects inefficiencies in the health care market. Economists have expressed two general reasons why the health care market may fail to reach an efficient outcome, or the optimal level of output where the marginal benefits of a good or service equal its marginal costs.[8,34]

First, health insurance interferes with the ability of the price system to allocate resources efficiently. In markets where consumers pay for goods and services directly, they generally balance the costs of what they purchase against the expected benefits. However, health insurance distorts this price signal, creating incentives for individuals to consume health care services that may be worth less to them than the full price of those services. Second, imperfect information among health care consumers may interfere with the efficient allocation of resources. Consumers of health care often lack full knowledge about the prices of different health care services, the quality of care offered by various providers, and the types and locations of alternative treatment products. This lack of information may affect demand and utilisation, and promote additional inefficiencies in the health care market.[21]

While some of the increase in health care spending may reflect market inefficiencies, much of the growth represents new benefits with substantial value to individuals, such as widespread access to technologies that improve patient outcome.[19,23] The basic question, therefore, is whether the growth is worth it: whether the value of the additional resources devoted to health care exceeds the benefits that could have been obtained by using those resources in alternative ways. That answer, however, depends on society's valuation of those benefits, as well as the overall willingness to trade-off additional spending on health care to direct productive resources into other goods and services.

ACCESS TO CARE AND THE UNINSURED

Access to health care has several dimensions: geographic location, the supply of providers, individual values about health and illness, the 'fit' between the patient seeking care and the provider, and the ability to pay for expected health care costs.[35] Access depends heavily on the last factor—ability to pay for care. For most Americans, that ability is secured through health insurance. Generally, the ability to pay is defined as financial access and is the focus of discussion in this section.

Major Sources of Health Insurance

The American health insurance system is based largely on a mix of public and private financing mechanisms that includes private group health insurance for workers and their dependants and public coverage for the elderly and certain categories of the poor and disabled. This public/private-based insurance system provides coverage to 212.8 million people, or 86% of the total population. The current arrangement, however, leaves 33.4 million uninsured, with relatively limited financial access to health care.[37] Before discussing this uninsured group, a brief overview of the major sources of health insurance and recent trends in coverage are presented as background for understanding the access issue.

Employment-based insurance

Health insurance as a benefit of employment has spread rapidly since the 1940s, when wartime price stabilisation policies froze wages and thus encouraged employers to offer health benefit packages to attract and retain workers.[38] These packages remain an attractive benefit to employees because they protect against the financial risk of medical expenses, and unlike cash compensation are tax-free. For the non-aged population, employer-based group health insurance is the single most important source of coverage. More than 150 million people under the age of 65, or about 70% of the non-elderly population, are covered by employment-related insurance, obtained either directly as a worker or as a dependant of a worker.[6]

While medium-to-large size firms traditionally have offered comprehensive health benefit packages to their workers, rising health care costs have prompted some smaller firms to limit coverage or eliminate health insurance for their workforce. A 1989 employer survey showed that only 33% of firms with fewer than ten employees offered health coverage, compared to almost all firms with 100 or more employees. The major reasons small firms gave for not providing coverage to their workers were high health insurance premiums and insufficient firm profits.[39,40]

Employer-based coverage in larger firms has also undergone some restructuring in coverage, scope of benefits and employees' share of insurance premiums. In 1980, about three-quarters (74%) of employees worked for firms that paid the full cost of individual coverage. By 1989, this figure had dropped to 55%. During this same period, the percentage of employees with no premium cost-sharing for family coverage dropped by 54% to 37%.[41] Additionally, some firms have reduced or eliminated coverage for pre-existing medical conditions or certain services (including substance abuse or psychiatric care), instituted extensive waiting periods following the beginning of employment, or implemented widespread cost-containment provisions. (e.g. almost 65% of Americans covered through the workplace have plans that include some type of pre-admission review programme to assess the 'appropriateness' or 'necessity' of hospitalization.)[42]

Medicare

Medicare, as a universal enfranchisement programme, is the principal source of coverage for the population age 65 and older. About 27 million, or 93% of the elderly, are insured through this programme, which also covers certain categories of non-elderly disabled people.[6]

Medicare has two separate components. Part A, the Hospital Insurance programme, provides basic protection against the costs of inpatient care and related basic post-hospital services for all persons aged 65 or older, certain categories of disabled individuals under age 65, and persons with end-stage renal disease. Part B, Supplementary Medical Insurance, is a voluntary programme for the aged and disabled that provides insurance benefits for physicians' services, laboratory testing, and outpatient hospital care. Almost all (95%) of the elderly chose to enroll in Medicare Part B coverage.

Of the four principal routes to coverage, 'Medicare has aged best', with the programme insuring more Americans each year for more acute care services.[43] There are, however, some gaps in coverage, and beneficiaries' out-of-pocket costs remain high. Medicare does not cover outpatient prescription drugs, for example, or most forms of preventive care, and limits some hospital and physician services. Protection against the costs of long-term care is also very slim, particularly with the repeal of the Medicare Catastrophic Act of 1988.

Medicaid

Medicaid is a federal/state entitlement programme that pays for medical services for low-income groups who also meet certain categorical requirements. Low-income groups eligible for the programme include pregnant women and children, the aged, and those with certain disabilities. About 14.6 million people, or 7% of the non-elderly population, are covered through the Medicaid programme.[6]

In contrast to Medicare, Medicaid coverage has eroded in recent years, in part due to the cost-containment initiatives of the early 1980s. Faced with growing Medicaid expenditures and decreased federal funds for the programme, several states have enacted arbitrary limits on basic services, such as the number of reimbursable hospital days and the frequency of physician visits. Eligibility requirements, however, were broadened in 1990, as Congress mandated the expansion of Medicaid coverage to pregnant women and young children up to 185% of the poverty level. Although it is too early to determine the impact of this mandate, historical trends show that the Medicaid programme has consistently failed to cover the majority of the population whose income and resources are insufficient to pay for health care. In 1983, it was estimated that Medicaid covered only 38.7% of the poverty population; by 1989, that figure had only risen to 40%.[43]

Other private insurance

Non-group, or 'self-purchased' health insurance, is available to individuals who are ineligible for the previous three routes to coverage. About 15 million people, or 7% of the non-elderly population, are insured through private, non-group policies.[6] The majority (64%) of these policies are purchased directly from commercial insurers and about one-third (29%) through Blue Cross/Blue Shield plans.[38]

Generally, self-purchased insurance is less comprehensive and more costly than employment-based coverage. Of the 15 million insured, some have only 'dread disease' coverage that provides limited benefits for specific illnesses; others have coverage limited to accidents or disabilities.[6] Further, some self-purchased policies include medical underwriting and either exclude coverage for certain pre-existing conditions contracted prior to enrolment or pay benefits only after a specified waiting period.[38] Privately purchased policies also typically have much higher administrative, or loading, costs than group-based plans. Loading costs for employment-based coverage in large firms (100 employees or more), for example, range from 6% to 16% of premiums; for self-purchased coverage, these costs are as high as 40% of premiums. Thus, individuals with self-purchased coverage pay more, on average, for the same scope of benefits, compared to those with group insurance plans.[6]

The Uninsured

Private and public health insurance coverage experienced rapid growth beginning in the 1940s, continuing through the 1960s with Medicare and Medicaid implementation. By the mid-1970s, however, this growth had ended, and a new trend—the erosion of insurance coverage as measured by the population insured—emerged in the 1980s. Data from the Current Population Survey conducted by the US Bureau of the Census, for example, show an overall growth in the number of uninsured, non-elderly Americans of about 8.4 million from 1979 to 1986.[38]

The increase in the proportion of people without insurance has been partially attributed to the economic recession of the early 1980s and the subsequent loss of employment-based coverage.[38] The economic recovery beginning in 1982, however, has not been met with a resultant decline in the percentage of the uninsured. The reasons for this are unclear. One possible explanation is that the post-1982 employment increases have been largely concentrated in the service industries, where employers are less likely to offer health insurance to their workers than in typical manufacturing industries. Other possible explanations for the growth include an overall movement away from employer-provided non-cash fringe benefits, changes in employer-sponsored health benefit plans that require greater employee cost sharing, and a decline in the population eligible for public programmes such as Medicaid.[44]

Estimates of the uninsured

Data from the March 1990 Current Population Survey (CPS) conducted by the US Bureau of the Census show that 33.4 million Americans lack public or private health insurance. The uninsured represent 13.6% of the total population and 15.3% of the population under age 65.[5] This estimate is considerably lower than the widely cited figure of 37.3 million found on the 1987 and earlier versions of the CPS. The difference between these estimates has been attributed to changes in the CPS survey design.[45]

Major changes in the CPS, including a reconstruction of the wording and sequence of the health insurance questions, were implemented in 1988. These changes, designed to improve the accuracy of health insurance coverage data and to gather new information about the coverage status of children, also resulted in lower estimates of the uninsured than those reported in earlier versions of the CPS. There is a general consensus among the research community that the lower estimate of 33.4 million reflects the improvements in survey questions, rather than a decline in the number of uninsured individuals.[44]

The underinsured

In addition to the uninsured, who have no financial protection from medical expenses, inadequate health care coverage, or underinsurance, leaves some people in private health plans at financial risk. 'Underinsurance', however, is not easily quantified and estimates of the number of uninsured individuals are difficult to develop. Population-based surveys on health insurance status, for example, generally do not reveal individual gaps in coverage for specific illnesses or medical conditions. Further, there is no standard definition of underinsurance. Some have defined the term based on a lack of coverage for particular types of care, such as preventive treatment or long-term care.[38] Others have defined underinsurance based on a specific dollar limit of uninsured health expenses (e.g. $15 000) or on the probability of incurring high out-of-pocket medical expenses relative to family income.[44]

Despite these difficulties, a 1985 study that accounted for a complexity of factors, including income, coverage provisions and expected levels of utilisation, estimated that 20 million privately-insured Americans under the age of 65 (or 12.6% of this population) were underinsured in 1988.[46] In other words, their private coverage left them open to a significant risk of spending 10% or more of their family income on medical expenses.[47] The poor and the near poor—and adults between the ages of 55 and 64—were most likely to have private coverage that left them vulnerable to this financial risk.

Characteristics of the uninsured

Certain groups—young adults, the poor and near-poor, and adults and children in families without an employed member—face greater than average risks of being uninsured. Young adults (between 18 and 24 years of age) are most likely to be uninsured; 25.1%, compared with the average rate of 13.6% for the population in 1990. In fact, about one-fifth (20.9%) of all adults under the age of 35 were uninsured in 1990. The risk of being uninsured decreases with age for the population age 35 and over, with only about 10.1% of men between the ages of 55 and 64 uninsured in 1990. Because of the near-universal coverage of those aged 65 and over through Medicare, only 1.0% of the elderly were uninsured in that year.[6]

Most of the uninsured are low income persons. In 1990, 28.8% had family incomes below the poverty level, and another 31.8% were near-poor (with incomes between 100–199% of the poverty level). About one-fifth (21.7%) of the uninsured had family incomes 300% or greater than the poverty level. The likelihood of being uninsured, however, is inversely related to income. Almost one-third (30.2%) of the poor and one-quarter (23.3%) of the near-poor were uninsured in 1990. By contrast, only about 6% of families with incomes of at least 300% of the poverty level were uninsured in that year.[6]

Although the majority (77.5%) of the uninsured are white, the risk of being uninsured is substantially higher for blacks and Hispanic Americans. In 1990, 19.2% of all blacks and 19.1% of all Hispanics were uninsured, compared with the rate of 12.5% among whites in that year.[6] About two-thirds of the uninsured live in the south (43.1%) and west (25.1%). The risk of being uninsured is also greater in these regions compared to the northeast and midwest regions.[45] Additionally, there are state-level coverage differences: the uninsured rate ranges from less than 10% in Massachusetts, Pennsylvania, Michigan,

Wisconsin and Iowa to more than 25% in Louisiana, Texas, and New Mexico.[48]

About one-half (47.1%) of the uninsured lived in two-parent families in 1990; single-parent families comprised another one-quarter (27.2%) of the uninsured population. The likelihood of being uninsured, however, varies substantially by family structure. Among children and adults living in single-parent families, 21.8% were uninsured in 1990, compared with 12.3% among two-parent families and only 6.3% among childless couples.[6]

Most of the uninsured (80.6%) have some connection to the workforce. In 1990, about 48.7% of the uninsured (under 65) population were either full-time or part-time workers, and another 31.9% were dependants of these workers. The number of hours worked by the head of household or spouse is closely related to the risk of being uninsured. About 34.2% of individuals in families with only part-time workers were uninsured in 1990, compared with 12.6% among those in families with at least one member who works full-time.[5]

Why the uninsured lack coverage

Access to employment-based coverage is the single most important factor that determines whether or not people have insurance. However, for some, particularly the working poor, insurance often is not available through their employer. Only about 43% of all firms, for example, offer insurance coverage to their workforce, according to a 1989 employer survey by the Health Insurance Association of America.[40] In general, workers who are not given insurance coverage by their employers are concentrated in the private sector and are more likely than their counterparts to be employed by smaller firms (25 employees or less), earning lower wages, and working on a part-time basis.[6,49]

Even when firms provide health insurance to their workforce, many employees remain uninsured, either because they are excluded from coverage or because they turn coverage down. More than two-thirds of all employers exclude part-time workers from their insurance plan; an estimated 13% of all workers do not accept employer-offered insurance. About one-half of these workers may turn down insurance because they are covered by a spouse's plan. However, the other half may turn down coverage because their share of the premium cost is prohibitive, based on their earnings and other family income.[44]

For many other low-income people, eligibility restrictions and enrolment difficulties prevent effective access to public insurance programmes. Medicaid eligibility, for example, is linked to both income standards and categorical requirements that exclude many of the uninsured from coverage, and the programme has consistently covered less than one-half of the poverty population.[50] Further, a substantial proportion of those individuals eligible for Medicaid do not enrol in the programme. One recent study estimated that only about 72% of those eligible for Medicaid assistance were enrolled in 1989.[44]

Possible reasons for the Medicaid enrolment shortfalls are numerous. Some individuals may not understand the programme eligibility requirements; others may be discouraged from enrolment due to the complex documentation and application process for coverage. Some eligible participants may not enrol because of difficulties in locating a provider who accepts Medicaid reimbursement. An estimated 25% of private practice physicians do not participate in the Medicaid programme, due to low reimbursement rates, extensive paperwork requirements, and lengthy payment delays.[44]

Individuals who are not offered employment-based coverage and who are not eligible for public programmes often cannot obtain self-purchased insurance at an affordable cost. As noted earlier, self-purchased insurance is relatively expensive, both because of the high administrative costs and because the plan premium is not shared with the employer. Further, people with pre-existing conditions, such as diabetes, heart disease, or AIDS, often are rejected as 'uninsurable' when they apply for coverage or they are required to pay substantially higher rates for their coverage.[6]

Health consequences

Lack of insurance coverage can affect individual health care utilisation and health status. The uninsured have been estimated to use 37% less physician services and 69% less hospital services than their insured counterparts.[51] Even when they are able to gain entry to the health care system, the uninsured may not fare as well as the insured in terms of treatment options and outcomes. A recent study found that people without insurance were less likely to receive routine diagnostic tests, less likely to undergo key surgical procedures (such as coronary bypass surgery and hip/knee replacements), and more likely to die during their hospital stay than those individuals with similar health status who had private insurance.[52] Although these results could be explained by factors other than the availability of insurance, they at least suggest that lack of coverage can make a significant difference in individual treatment options and health outcomes.

CONCLUSION

The rising concern over reform of the US health care system has been fuelled by continued growth in health care spending and the large number of Americans without health insurance coverage. These problems and their causes are well documented, yet a consensus on policy solutions has proved elusive. This irresolution may continue, given the divergent political, cultural and interest-group forces that have shaped the American health care system. Acceptance of cost-control mechanisms such as fixed budgets for health expenditures used in Canada and Western European nations would appear unlikely in the USA because this 'would imply the acceptance of a philosophy of limits—an enormously difficult concept to sell in light of our material abundance, our fascination with technology and our resistance to the imposition of constraints'.[53]

Health reform advocates will undoubtedly continue to offer

alternative policy solutions to expand access and control health expenditures, ensuring a prominent position for health reform on the national agenda. However, it is a consensus position among the myriad of currently proposed reform strategies—and one that addresses the concerns of government, business, providers and consumers regarding the financing and delivery of health care—that would prove far more useful towards strengthening the American health care system.

ACKNOWLEDGEMENTS

The author gratefully acknowledges the assistance of John C. Gaffney and Edward B. Hirshfeld for comments and suggestions, and Mary Ann Ohms for research assistance.

REFERENCES

1. Blendon, R., Leitman, R., Morrison, I. and Donelan, K. Satisfaction with health systems in ten nations. *Health Affairs* 1990; **9(2)**: 185–192.
2. *Comparing Health Systems: Health Service Satisfaction in Six Countries*, Boston, Harvard Community Health Plan and Louis Harris & Associates, 1990.
3. Levit, K., Lazenby, H., Letsch, S. and Cowan, C. National health spending, 1989. *Health Affairs* 1991; **10(1)**: 117–130.
4. Schieber, G. and Poullier, J. International health spending: issues and trends. *Health Affairs* 1991; **10(1)**: 106–116.
5. Congressional Budget Office. *Rising Health Care Costs: Causes, Implications and Strategies*, Washington, DC, Government Printing Office, 1991.
6. Congressional Budget Office. *Selected Options for Expanding Health Insurance Coverage*. Washington, DC, Government Printing Office, 1991.
7. Levit, K., Freeland, M. and Waldo, D. National health care spending trends: 1988. *Health Affairs* 1990; **9(2)**: 171–184.
8. *Medicare and the American Health Care System*, Washington, DC, Prospective Payment Assessment Commission, June 1991.
9. Congressional Budget Office. *Trends in Health Care Expenditures by*

Medicare and the Nation. Washington, DC, Government Printing Office, 1991.
10. Comparisons of international spending data are subject to some methodological difficulties because countries do not use standard definitions and service accounts to determine health expenditures. Practices of reporting mortality statistics such as infant mortality and cause-specific death rates may also vary significantly among countries. (See Schieber, G. and Poullier, J., ref. 4, for a full description of such variations.)
11. Gross domestic product (GDP) equals gross national product less net property income from abroad. GDP is used in international comparisons of health spending because it corrects for variations in the role of foreign transactions in different economies.
12. Aaron, H. A prescription for health care. In: Aaron H. (ed.) *Setting National Priorities*, Washington, DC, Brookings Institution, 1990.
13. Fuchs, V. *Who Shall Live*. New York, Basic Books, 1983.
14. *CPI Detailed Report 16*. Washington, DC, Bureau of Labor Statistics, US Department of Labor, December 1990.
15. Fuchs, V. The 'competitive revolution' in health care. *Health Affairs*. 1988; **7(2)**: 5–24.
16. Baumol, W. Containing medical costs: why price controls won't work. *Public Interest* 1988; **93**: 37–53.
17. Newhouse, J. Measuring medical prices and understanding their effects: the Baxter Foundation prize address. *Journal of Health Administration Education* 1989; **7**: 19–26.
18. Pauly, M. Taxation, health insurance, and market failure in the medical economy. *Journal of Economic Literature* 1986; **24**: 629–675.
19. Aaron, H. and Schwartz, W. Rationing health care: the choice before us. *Science*. 1990; **247**: 418–423.
20. Aaron, H. *Serious and Unstable Condition: Financing America's Health Care*. Washington, DC, Brookings Institution, 1991.
21. Feldstein, P. *Health Care Economics*. 2nd edn, New York, Wiley, 1983.
22. Arno, P., Shenson, D., Siegel, N., Franks, P. and Lee, P. Economic and policy implications of early intervention in HIV disease. *Journal of the American Medical Association* 1989; **262**: 1493–1498.
23. Fuchs, V. The health sector's share of the gross national product, *Science* 1990; **247**: 534–538.
24. Waldo, D., Sonnefeld, S., McKusick, D. and Arnett, R. Health expenditures by age group, 1977 and 1987. *Health Care Financing Review* 1989; **10(4)**: 116–118.
25. Lubitz, J. and Prihoda, R. The use and costs of Medicare services

in the last 2 years of life. *Health Care Financing Review* 1984; **5(3)**: 117–131.
26. Center for Health Policy Research. *The Cost of Medical Professional Liability in the 1980s*, Chicago, American Medical Association, 1990.
27. Coddington, D., Keen, D., Moore, K. and Clarke, R. *The Crisis in Health Care*, San Francisco, Jossey-Bass, 1990.
28. Levit, K., Lazenby, H., Cowan, C. and Letsch, S. National health expenditures, 1990. *Health Care Financing Review* 1991; **13(1)**: 29–55.
29. Democratic Study Group. *Why Conservatives Don't Talk About America's Health System*, No. 102–6, May 24, 1991.
30. Battistella, R. and Weil, T. National health insurance reconsidered: dilemmas and opportunities. *Hospital and Health Services Administration*. 1989; **34**: 139–156.
31. *Survey of Current Business*. Washington, DC: Bureau of Economic Analysis, US Department of Commerce; July 1990; and Health Care Financing Administration, National Health Accounts, unpublished data, 1991.
32. Reinhart, U. Health care spending and American competitiveness. *Health Affairs*. 1989; **8(4)**: 4–21.
33. Fraser, D. A national health policy debate. *Dartmouth Medical School Alumni Magazine* Summer 1989; 30.
34. Gramlich, E. *Benefit–Cost Analysis of Government Programs*. Englewood Cliffs, NJ, Prentice-Hall, 1981.
35. Brown, E. Access to health insurance in the United States. *Medical Care Review* 1989; **46**: 349–385.
36. Unless otherwise noted, population estimates noted herein on the number and percentage of the population covered by various public and private insurance plans are based on Congressional Budget Office estimates from the March 1990 Current Population Survey.
37. Statement of Robert D. Reischauer, Director, Congressional Budget Office, before the House Committee on Ways and Means, 102nd Congress, 1st Session, 23 April 1991.
38. Congressional Research Service. *Health Insurance and the Uninsured: Background Data and Analysis*. Washington, DC, Government Printing Office, 1988.
39. *Health Insurance: Cost Increases Lead to Coverage Limitations and Cost Shifting*, Washington, DC, US General Accounting Office, 1990. HRD-90-68.
40. *Providing Employee Health Benefits: How Firms Differ*. Washington, DC, Health Insurance Association of America, 1990.
41. *Employee Benefits in Medium and Large Firms, 1988*. Washington,

DC, Bureau of Labor Statistics, US Department of labor, 1989. Bulletin 2336.
42. Gabel, J., DiCarlo, S., Fink, S. and de Lissovoy, G. Employer-sponsored health insurance in America. *Health Affairs* 1989; **8(2)**: 116–128.
43. Friedman, E. The uninsured: from dilemma to crisis. *Journal of the American Medical Association* 1991; **265**: 2491–2495.
44. Lewin/ICF. *The Health Care Financing System and the Uninsured*. Submitted to the Office of Research, Health Care Financing Administration, US Department of Health and Human Services, December 22, 1989.
45. Moyer, E. A revised look at the number of uninsured Americans. *Health Affairs*. 1989; **8(2)**: 102–110.
46. Farley, P. Who are the uninsured? *Milbank Memorial Fund Quarterly* 1985; **63**: 476–503.
47. This figure represents the proportion of the privately insured who had a 1% or greater risk of incurring out-of-pocket medical expenses in excess of 10% of their family income.
48. Chollet, D., Foley, J. and Mages, C. *Uninsured in the USA: The Nonelderly Population Without Health Insurance, 1988*, Washington, DC, Employee Benefit Research Institute, 1990.
49. Short, P., Monheit, A. and Beauregard, K. *National Medical Expenditure Survey: A Profile of Uninsured Americans: Research Findings 1*. Rockville, MD, National Center for Health Services Research and Health Care Technology Assessment; 1990.
50. Swartz, K. and Lipson, D. *Strategies for Assisting the Medically Uninsured*. Washington, DC, Urban Institute and the Intergovernmental Health Policy Project, 1989.
51. Long, S. and Rodgers, J. *The Effects of Being Uninsured on Health Care Service Use Estimates from the Survey of Income and Program Participation*, Washington, DC, US Bureau of the Census; 1990. SIPP Working Paper No. 9012.
52. Hadley, J., Steinberg, E. and Feder, J. Comparison of uninsured and privately insured hospital patients: conditions on admission, resource use and outcome. *Journal of the American Medical Association* 1991; **265**: 374–379.
53. Levy, S. and Hill, J. National health insurance: the triumph of equivocation. *New England Journal of Medicine* 1989; **321**: 1750–1754.

CHAPTER 9

Proposals to reform the US health care system: a critical review*

John C. Gaffney,
Susan M. Browning and
Edward B. Hirshfeld
American Medical Association,
Chicago, Illinois, USA

INTRODUCTION

A variety of factors suggests that fundamental reform of the US health care system could be implemented in the near future. First, proposals to restructure the US health care system have proliferated rapidly. This proliferation reflects growing support for the view that health system reform is necessary and has become politically feasible. Second, calls for health system reform are emanating from mainstream groups, such as organised medicine, business, labour, political leaders, and governmental commissions. Third, the media are devoting an increasing amount of attention to problems in health care and the need for reforms. Fourth, attitudinal surveys find strong public support for implementing major changes in the US

* The views expressed in this chapter are those of the authors and may not represent those of the American Medical Association.

North American Health Care Policy in the 1990s
Edited by A. King, T. Hyclak, S. McMahon and R. Thornton

health care system. Fifth, health reform was one of the points of contention between the Republicans and Democrats in the 1992 election campaigns. Calls by Democratic presidential candidates for health reforms forced the Bush Administration to undertake the development of its own health reform proposal. By mid-1992, both major political parties appeared to be committed to implementing some sort of health system reform.

Although broad agreement seems to exist on the need for reform, a consensus does not exist on what changes should be made. Differences among reform proposals are large because general agreement does not yet exist on answers to basic questions such as: what goals should society set for the health care sector; what is the optimal trade-off among those goals; what economic philosophy should govern the production and distribution of health care; and what are the appropriate roles and responsibilities of governments, businesses, third parties, providers and patients in the health care sector? To some, this situation suggests that significant health system reform is unlikely in the near future. History provides some support for this view since the USA appeared to be on the verge of implementing national health insurance (NHI) in the late 1940s and again in the early 1970s but political support for NHI proved insufficient. However, the current environment in which health system reform is being considered may be significantly different from that of previous eras. Specifically, the health care cost problem—high and rapidly rising health care prices and expenditures—appears to be much larger and more serious today. Spokespersons for governments, business and even health care provider groups have repeatedly stated that current trends in health care costs are unsustainable and that rising health care expenditures threaten the viability of other governmental programmes and the international competitiveness of US business. Unlike previous eras, provider groups that have traditionally opposed governmental attempts to restructure the health sector are now actively advocating health system reform because, in part, they believe that a government-controlled health care system (such as exists in Canada and the UK) is inevitable unless the rate of increase in US health care expenditures is reduced.

The purpose of this chapter is to provide a critical review of the current discussion of health system reform in the USA. The first section outlines a framework that can be used to analyse reform proposals. The second section uses that analytical framework to provide a critical review of a selected set of reform proposals. The chapter concludes with discussions of the basic choices that are being offered by the current set of reform proposals and the political prospects for health system reform in the USA

DEFINITION AND FRAMEWORK FOR ANALYSIS

The meaning of the term 'health system reform' is somewhat ambiguous. In recent decades, the US health sector has seen the emergence of new delivery systems, the growth and decline of multi-hospital systems, hospital closures in rural and inner city areas, the growth of group practice, increased intrusion by third parties into clinical decision-making, rapid increases in malpractice claims and costs, and changes in Medicare payment systems for hospitals and physicians. The cumulative effect of these changes is substantial; the US health care system in the early 1990s differs in significant ways from that of the early 1970s. However, the rhetoric surrounding the current debate suggests that what is meant by 'health system reform' is something different from the evolutionary changes that have occurred over the past two decades.

What is apparently meant by health system reform is enactment of a major legislative package that has the objective of causing changes in the institutional or economic structure of the health sector to induce a significant change in performance of the sector and place it on a different evolutionary path. (This definition follows the paradigm that an industry's structure determines its conduct which, in turn, determines its performance.) Using this definition, at least three reformations of the

US health care sector can be identified. First, the passage of medical practice acts and legislation prohibiting the corporate practice of medicine by state governments in the late nineteenth and early twentieth centuries established the legal and institutional framework for medical practice in the USA. Second, the passage of the Hill-Burton Act in the 1950s led to rapid growth in the number of hospitals, which in turn led to rapid development and diffusion of expensive medical technologies, growth in hospital-based specialties, and more pervasive and objective quality-assurance mechanisms. Third, the establishment of the Medicare and Medicaid programmes in the mid-1960s increased access to and demand for medical care, greatly expanded the role of governments in health care, and contributed significantly to the escalation of health care prices and expenditures.

The debate over health system reform is also confused by the way the reform proposals are presented. Proponents of health system reform usually do not clearly articulate the assumptions, goals and values of their proposals. Most reform proposals highlight their strengths, but are silent about potential weaknesses and adverse effects. Further, all of the current proposals are incomplete in the sense that they do not provide a full picture of how the proposed new health system will function.

An analytical framework that sets out a common format and vocabulary is needed to facilitate comparison and evaluation of the various reform proposals. The framework proposed below begins with a set of broad questions to ask about any proposal.

Broad Questions

Seven broad questions should be posed for any reform proposal. They are:

1. What goals for the health care system are identified and prioritised?
2. What failures of the current health system are identified?

3. What causes are identified as being responsible for the failures?
4. What paradigms and values provide the foundation of the proposal?
5. How would the proposal affect key aspects of the health care system?
6. What are the likely social trade-offs that would result from implementation of the proposal?
7. What is the political feasibility of the proposal?

Goals

The first step is to identify the goals that the proposal sets for the health sector and the priorities that it establishes for those goals. Identifying the goals and priorities can be difficult because some proposals do not explicitly state them.

The goals established for the health sector by any reform proposal can be organised into two categories—generally accepted societal goals and goals specific to the interest group which developed the proposal. Traditionally, three broad societal goals are endorsed for the US health care sector: (i) a 'reasonable' and 'acceptable' level of health care costs; (ii) an acceptable level of quality of the health care product; and (iii) an acceptable level of access to the health care product. These goals are often described by the short hand phrase 'cost, quality, and access'.

Although the cost–quality–access goals are widely accepted, they are usually not carefully defined or justified—a situation that also contributes to confusion. At various times, discussions of the cost goal have focused on all of the following: percentage of gross domestic product (GDP) allocated to health care, per capita and average family expenditures on health care, the ratio of corporate outlays for health benefits to corporate profits, and the price of the health care 'product'. Concern about rising health care costs (however defined) is understandable if, as is widely believed, the rapid rise in costs is due to rampant economic inefficiency in the health care sector but, the concept of a health care cost goal seems to relate to target levels. For example, forecasts that health care will 'consume' over 20% of the US GDP early in the next century have usually been followed by the comment that the USA cannot afford that level of health spending. Some US Congressmen have begun to discuss strategies to stabilise health spending at 15–16% of GDP as if the USA could afford no more than that level of spending. The perception that seems to underlie the concept of a target level of health care spending is that health care is somehow different from other products—health care is a 'drag' on the economy—and that society can afford only so much of it.

Great debate exists about how to define and measure quality—input characteristics, process or outcomes. Less debate exists about the concept that the quality of health care (however defined) should not fall below a target level or that quality should vary within a narrow range. That quality standards must be maintained or increased is almost an article of faith among US physicians. Attitudinal surveys suggest that the US public believes that the quality of health care should not fall below some target level and that large variations in the quality of health care should not exist across classes of patients (high income versus low income).

The explanation for a goal of limited variation in the quality of health care is not entirely obvious. One possible justification is that health care is so technically complex that consumers must use agents (physicians) to help them make consumption decisions, and that the concept that quality should vary within a narrow range arose as a mechanism to prevent physicians from taking advantage of their positions by delivering low-quality care but charging for high-quality care. Another possible justification is that health care consumption decisions must frequently be made under situations of emotional stress, making rational decisions about quality difficult. Thus society evolved a convention of limiting variations in the quality of health care to a narrow range to help consumers approximate rational decision-making.

Perhaps the most likely explanation for a quality goal relates to the perceived linkage between the quality and quantity of health care consumed and the continued existence of the patient. The linkage between health care consumption and human life makes access to and quality of medical care highly value-laden issues for most Americans. This situation can probably be traced to the Judaeo-Christian religious foundations for much of American culture and law. As evidenced by the history of legal prohibitions in the USA against abortion and suicide, and the current vitriolic debate over abortion, many US residents view human life as sacred, with a value that is perhaps immeasurable in economic terms. Consequently, the concept that the quality of health care should fall below a given level may have evolved as a mechanism to prevent patients from choosing a quality level that is associated with a high risk of death.

Discussions of access to health care seem to have three components: the total supply and geographic distribution of health care resources, non-economic barriers to health care technologies (e.g. regulations that require governmental approval of drugs and devices), and financial barriers that limit consumption of health care services. Since a significant portion of the US population (about 13%) has no health care insurance coverage, the current discussion of health system reform focuses almost exclusively on financial barriers that limit consumption of health care. The access goal seems to be that every American should have the potential to consume at least a target quantity of health care. That goal is usually articulated as a requirement that every American have a health insurance policy (or health benefit plan) that covers 'basic' health care services with low (20% or lower) co-payments.

The explanation for a social goal of ensuring that every American has the financial potential to consume at least a target quantity of health care is probably the perceived linkage between health care consumption and life, as discussed above. Support for this argument is provided by the widespread view that physicians and hospitals have a moral obligation to provide charity care to the poor and needy. But the explanation for an access goal probably goes beyond the linkage between health care consumption and life because very little consideration is being given to permitting wealthy and high-income individuals to 'opt out' and not carry health insurance. The idea that everyone, including the wealthy, should have a basic health plan probably is an attempt to reduce the problems and inequities that arise from shifting the costs of uncompensated care to those who do have health insurance.

Another possible explanation for an access goal is the similarities between health care and education. Like education, consumption of health care services often enhances human capital, increasing the individual's ability to generate income and also increasing the individual's ability to enjoy a given level of consumption of goods and services. The similarities between the education product and the health product may be significant since the USA has made a commitment to ensure that every individual has access to a basic education without regard to ability to pay.

Although the cost–quality–access goals are generally accepted for the health sector, they are quite unusual when viewed from the perspective of other sectors of the US economy. Society's primary goal for most sectors of the economy is economic efficiency—production and distribution of the product with the least cost combination of resources. In a free market system, vigorous economic competition is the prescription for achieving economic efficiency. Consequently, endorsement of the cost, quality and access goals for the health sector implies that the health care product has some unique characteristics and that laissez-faire economic competition is unlikely to achieve society's goals for the health sector.

Health reform proposals differ somewhat in the extent to which they accept the traditional cost–quality–access goals, how they define the goals, and the priorities they place on them. Nevertheless, all of the major proposals identify expanding access and containing costs as high-priority goals.

Most of the current reform proposals have been developed by interest groups and, consequently, emphasise somewhat self-serving goals. For example, a reform proposal developed by health insurers may include an implicit goal of maintaining a role for private health insurance companies in the new health care system. A physician association may want to preserve or enhance clinical and economic autonomy for physicians. Business groups may want to reduce their expenses related to providing health care benefits to employees. Consumer groups may want to maximise access and minimise out-of-pocket costs for their members.

Failures

The second step in evaluating a reform proposal is to identify the perceived failures of the current system. The failures mentioned generally reflect the goals endorsed by the authors of the proposal. As with the goals, the perceived failures may be those generally agreed upon by society, or they may relate to the interests of a particular interest group.

Almost all reform proposals mention two failures: (i) limited access to health care services by segments of the population because of financial barriers; and (ii) unacceptably high levels of expenditures on health care. Aspects of these problems which are frequently mentioned include: racial inequality in access to health care services; high rates of increase in health care prices and expenditures; a low ratio of benefit to cost for some health care services; and a low level of production efficiency in the health care sector.

As is the case with health goals, agreement does not exist about which failures are the most important to correct. Perceptions about which failure is the most serious are also influenced by how interest groups are affected by different failures.

Causes

The third step in evaluating a reform proposal is to identify the specific causes which are blamed for the failures of the current system to achieve the desirable health goals. Some of the failures are viewed as contributing to other failures. For example, rising health care prices are frequently seen as contributing to decreasing access to health care services. However, a wide range of other causal factors are frequently mentioned, including: too little or too much economic competition; too little or too much governmental interference in the health sector; too much interference by third parties in clinical decision-making; excessively complex health benefit programmes; excessive diffusion of expensive medical technologies; attenuation of incentives to economise because of overly generous health insurance coverage; economic incentives that encourage physicians and others to provide too much care; and demographic changes in the general population.

Paradigms and Values

The fourth, and probably most difficult, step is to identify the paradigms and values that provide the foundation for the reform proposal. (Logically, this step should be the first one; but inferences about paradigms and values usually cannot be made until the analysis of goals, failures and causes is completed.) Values and ethics underlie the societal goals for the health care system and the failures that society currently perceives. The economic interests of various groups and other self-interests also play a role, but they are balanced with broader values and ethics. Interest groups usually try to rationalise their self-interested goals in terms of the ethics and values of society.

With regard to paradigms, the starting point is to ask whether the authors of the proposal see the health care product as having characteristics that are uniquely different from those of other products. If they do not, their reform proposal is likely to emphasise restructuring the health sector such that it approximates a freely competitive market. Recommended policies are likely to include the dismantling of governmental health regulations, programmes, planning, and possibly even loosening of licensing standards for health professionals and facilities. With the possible exception of the proposal of the

Heritage Foundation, all of the major reform proposals seem to accept the view that the health care product has some unique characteristics.

Much of the debate about health system reform involves disagreements about how much deviation from the pure competition model is needed to achieve society's goals for the health sector. At one extreme are those who emphasise individual responsibility, individual freedom, and free competition as the best form of economic organisation to meet the needs of the individual. Those who endorse this view usually argue that only minor interventions into the health care market are needed. At the other extreme are proponents of social responsibility, limitations on economic freedom, and centralised planning to meet individual needs. These individuals usually see only a limited role for market forces in the health sector.

The delivery of health care presents an ethical problem for both of the camps. If individual responsibility and free competition are relied upon to allocate health care, it is inevitable that some individuals will not be able to purchase the health care product and will, as a consequence, lose the enjoyment of life or life itself. If life is sacred or has a value that is immeasurable in economic terms, proponents of the competitive paradigm have an unresolved ethical dilemma. They also have to explain why almost every other developed country has chosen to reject the pure competition model for health care.

Those that totally reject the competitive paradigm have the problem of justifying why the costs of individual decisions to live unhealthy or risky lifestyles should be imposed on society. They also have to justify the cost to society of additional economic inefficiency (including the excess burden of additional taxes) that is inevitable if competitive forces are significantly attenuated and governments use regulation to direct the production and distribution of the health care product. Paradoxically, rejection of the competitive paradigm can lead to underfunding of health care systems and to non-market rationing of health care services. Advocates of centralised planning often justify non-market rationing on the grounds that health care will be distributed equitably.

Most health reform proposals advocate a blend of government intervention and market forces in the health care sector. These proposals are difficult to sort out because the differences in underlying values and goals are more subtle, and the influences of various paradigms about economic behaviour are less clear.

Differentiating between proposals that are advocated by groups with economic interests in the health system and those that are advanced by academics or institutions with particular value systems or political philosophies can be useful in identifying the extent to which pure values as opposed to economic interests provide the foundation of a reform proposal.

Potentially useful questions to pose include the following:

1. What perspective do the proponents have on the importance of individual responsibility, economic freedom and free competition as opposed to the value of social responsibility to the individual?
2. How strongly do the proponents feel about the need to maintain equality of access to health care services—do they believe in absolute equality (as in Canada where individuals with the same medical conditions have exactly the same potential command over health care resources regardless of their personal income or wealth levels) or are differentials acceptable once a certain level of equality of access is achieved (as in the US Medicare system where individuals can choose to purchase supplemental health insurance)?
3. What value do the advocates place on the quality of health care services and facilitating medical progress in comparison to other values, such as equality?
4. How important is production efficiency and control over health care prices and expenditures to the advocates, and what values are they willing to compromise to gain control?
5. What paradigms of economic behaviour do the advocates believe in, and how is the proposal structured around these paradigms?

Effects on Key Components of the Health Sector

The fifth step is to evaluate how effective a reform proposal would be in resolving perceived problems with the health care system. The assessment should consider the following:

1. Whether the reforms being advocated would be effective in resolving the identified problems. For example, if the proposal is primarily concerned with assuring universal access to health care, the mechanisms that it proposes need to be evaluated to determine how effective they would be in achieving that goal.
2. Whether the proposal is sufficiently comprehensive. The evaluation should determine whether the proposal considers and has methods for resolving problems that its advocates are not primarily concerned about, but which need to be addressed if the reform is to be implementable. For example, if a proposal is primarily concerned with assuring access, it is important to evaluate whether it also proposes effective methods to control costs without compromising quality.
3. Whether the proposal has anticipated and has solutions for problems that its methods might create with the functioning of key components of the health care system. For example, if the proposal would control costs by imposing price controls on providers, how would the proposal prevent the controls from causing adverse effects on supply or quality?

A systemic way to evaluate the effectiveness of a proposal is to consider its effect on the key functions or components of a health care system. The impact of the proposal on the following areas should be considered: (a) coverage criteria, (b) scope of benefits, (c) costs, (d) sources of financing, (e) payer responsibility, (f) administration, (g) cost control, (h) quality assurance, (i) recruitment and payment of providers, (j) recruitment and payment of suppliers of medical goods and equipment, (k) education of health care professionals, and (l) financing for research and development of new technology.

For example, focusing on coverage criteria reveals how well a proposal assures access. A proposal may purport to assure that all citizens have access to care but then set criteria for participation in subsidised health plans at income levels that are unrealistically low. Or, a proposal may provide for universal access to government-funded health care plans with no coverage criteria, but the scope of benefits might be too restrictive to provide many types of essential health care. A systematic appraisal of the effects of health care plans on these key functions and components of a health care system makes it possible to evaluate the impact of each proposal as a whole, and makes it possible to compare them to each other. The evaluation and comparison will reveal which proposals make a serious effort to effectively address the perceived problems of the health care system in a complete and practical fashion. It will also reveal the trade-offs that each proposal makes in order to achieve its primary goal, which makes it possible for individuals to judge which trade-offs most completely match their own ethics and values.

Social Trade-offs

The sixth step in analysing a reform proposal is to try to identify the social trade-offs that are inherent in the proposal. All of the proposals, at least implicitly, propose some change in the trade-off among health sector goals. Indeed, much of what is currently being called health system reform may be nothing more than attempts to change the current trade-off among society's goals for the health sector.

A trade-off among health goals is probably unavoidable because the goals are, to some extent, incompatible with each other. For example, emphasising access and high quality is likely to imply ineffective control over prices and expenditures. Similarly, emphasising access and control over expenditures is likely to imply reductions in quality standards.

A lack of appreciation for the inherent trade-off among health goals may explain some of the historical dynamics of the health sector. Concern about quality standards in the early part of the century led to closure of medical schools and hospitals and, after World War II, to expanding government support for medical research. As quality levels rose, access became a more serious problem. Concerns about access in the 1950s and 1960s led to governmental programmes to encourage the development of hospitals and to provide health benefit coverage to the elderly and poor. Advances in medical technology and expansion in access set the stage for the cost increases that characterised the 1970s and 1980s. Cost increases over the past decade have, in turn, exacerbated the access problem.

Questions that could be posed about trade-offs include the following. Does the proposal explicitly recognise trade-offs among goals? What is the recommended trade-off and how would it affect participants in the health sector? Does the proposal recommend improving economic efficiency as a way to avoid the trade-off problem? Does the proposal offer a socially acceptable, stable equilibrium among health goals?

Feasibility

The final step is to assess the political feasibility of the reform proposal. In general, the more complex a proposal and the larger the proposed changes in current roles and responsibilities, the lower the political feasibility of that proposal. The proposals that focus on arcane changes in federal tax policy or the national health insurance proposals that depend on expansion in taxes and government bureaucracy are likely to have a low level of political feasibility because Americans generally have a low level of trust in the ability of their governments to manage economic programmes.

The reactions of providers and interest groups must be considered because they are capable of mounting substantial opposition to a particular proposal. The proposals, for example, that include the elimination of the private health insurance industry are likely to have a low level of feasibility. Finally, the degree to which a proposal appears to offer the public what it wants should be considered. Attitudinal surveys suggest that the public will support reform proposals that appear to offer universal health benefit coverage with low out-of-pocket costs for that coverage, strong controls on health care prices, freedom of choice of provider, low out-of-pocket costs for the consumer of health care services, and limited or no tax increases. Strong public support would probably exist for requiring employers to finance benefit plans covering 'necessary' medical care services, low or non-existent deductibles and co-insurance rates for consumers of 'necessary' health care services, and the imposition of price controls on the health care sector.

REVIEW AND ANALYSIS OF MAJOR PROPOSALS

This section provides a critical review of five reform proposals that have been selected to illustrate the range of approaches that are being considered under the rubric of health system reform. The reviews are the result of applying the analytic framework developed above.

The Heritage Foundation Proposal

The Heritage proposal was developed by conservative economists who believe that market forces should govern health care.[1] It is meant to provide universal access while approximating a market as closely as possible.

Underlying goals and values

The goals of the proposal include (i) universal access, (ii) improvement of the efficiency of the health care system, (iii) moderation of cost escalations in health care, and (iv) reduction of the burden of health care costs on the overall economy. The primary underlying values are (a) individual freedom, especially freedom of choice, (b) individual responsibility, and (c) concern over the fairness of requiring an individual to pay for the health care of another. These values are balanced by compassion for the individual who may die or become disabled without access to health care, or who may face catastrophic financial losses due to health care problems that are not within the individual's control.

The proposal falls short of recommending complete reliance on market forces to guide the distribution of health care in order to accommodate the value of compassion for individuals who would lose access as a result. However, the proposal never explains why full application of market forces would be incompatible with this basic value.

Perception of the problem

The Heritage economists believe that two factors are the basis for the problems with the health care system being experienced today: (i) favourable tax treatment for employer provided health plans, and (ii) weak incentives for beneficiaries of those plans to make cost-effective decisions about health care consumption. The favourable tax treatment has resulted in widespread use of employer-based plans and has encouraged individuals to 'over-insure', thereby contributing to escalating health care expenditures. The Heritage Foundation believes the current health care system will eventually become non-viable as cost increases make it impossible for business and government to provide adequate health plans to large segments of the population.

The proposal argues that the current system cannot be salvaged with marginal adjustments, and must be replaced with a system that revitalises market forces. Mandated employer-provided health plans are rejected as likely to increase labour costs to the point that labour markets are adversely affected. Additionally, the proposal argues that Canadian-style national health insurance would cause a chronic imbalance between supply and demand, price and budget controls, and non-market rationing of health care.

Elements of the proposal

Universal access would be achieved by legislating that each household acquire a health plan with benefits that meet or exceed a prescribed benefits package. Tax credits would help defray the cost of health plans and the purchase of medical services. The credit amount would depend on the ratio of family out-of-pocket spending on health care to its income. The higher the ratio, the higher the percentage of spending that would qualify for the credit. Employer-provided health plans would count as taxable income to the employee. Employers that eliminate health plans would be required to distribute the value of the benefits as income to employees. Employers could act as negotiating agents for employees to help them secure health insurance coverage at favourable rates.

Medicare would be restructured. To alter consumption incentives, Medicare taxes and premiums paid by the elderly would be abolished, and deductibles and co-payments would be increased. Alternatively, beneficiaries could elect to receive a Medicare voucher which could be used to purchase a government-approved health plan. Beneficiaries could supplement the voucher with their own money to buy expensive plans, or they could buy an economical plan for less than the voucher and keep the difference. Tax credits would also be used to encourage individuals to fund health care savings accounts, which would function like health care individual retirement accounts (IRAs).

The poor would continue to be covered by Medicaid, although states would have more freedom to experiment with financing and delivery methods. States would be encouraged to develop risk pools for uninsurable individuals and to develop catastrophe plans for families threatened with bankruptcy due to medical expenses.

Incentives would be established to encourage individuals to purchase long-term care insurance. A new federal and state long-term care programme would be created for low-income individuals.

Trade-offs

While the proposal attempts to provide for universal access, that goal is compromised by its reliance on market forces. Most middle class families would find increased financial barriers to consuming health care. Those barriers are essential to the proposal because they would be relied upon to ignite competitive forces as families search for affordable plans and affordable care. In addition, the design of the Medicare, Medicaid, long-term care, risk pools and catastrophe plans does not guarantee access for the elderly, poor, uninsurable and victims of catastrophic expenses.

The proposal leaves quality of care to be regulated by the market. That approach would probably result in lower quality levels because consumers will have difficulty paying for high-quality care and may also defer consumption of preventive care and necessary care. No attention is given to regulating incentives for plans to withhold care in order to conserve costs in the race to be more competitive.

The growth of managed care systems that would result from implementation of the Heritage proposal would probably reduce physicians' clinical autonomy. Managed care plans are likely to seek additional control over physician decision making as a strategy to make themselves more price competitive. In addition, no tort reform measures are suggested to address the problem of 'defensive medicine' that results from judicial regulation of physicians.

Reliance on market forces might adversely affect the rate at which medical technology advances as no provisions are made for government funding of research and development. Although substantial externalities are associated with technological advances in health care, the proposal would limit the government's role to monitoring the market, subsidising the individual, and encouraging competition.

One trade-off is left unexplained. The proposal would

require open enrolment and community rating for health plans that cover Medicare beneficiaries, but not for plans that cover the rest of the population. The rejection of open enrolment and community rating is one reason why the plan must provide for risk pools and catastrophe plans. The reasons for this decision are not clear.

Feasibility

The feasibility of the Heritage proposal is low. Business interests would support the plan because it promises to lower their health outlays. But the typical voter is likely to find the requirement that individuals be responsible for their own health plans to be threatening. They will be doubtful that the promised tax credits and deductions will be sufficient to fund a good health insurance plan. Labour will also oppose the loss of an important employer-provided benefit. Some physicians will favour the proposal because of the promise of additional autonomy. But other physicians will oppose it because of the likely increase in managed care systems and because of the potential for degradation of quality levels.

Comment and summary

The proposal is creative and thought-provoking, although not feasible. It is so revolutionary that many institutions and methods of operation would be eliminated or changed dramatically. Therein lies the most important conceptual weaknesses of the proposal. It fails to explain how some key functions would be handled. For example, it does not anticipate how prices would be set in the context of market forces or what would be done with many of the existing price controls. It also fails to consider or address how to account for many of the effects of the changes that would result, some of which may be adverse. A good example is the failure to consider or account for the potential adverse effects on quality and the likelihood that there will continue to be uninsured individuals.

One strength of the proposal is its recognition that the

current health care system is probably misallocating scarce resources and reducing the international competitiveness of American business. It also recognises that a minimum wage combined with mandated employer-provided health plans would continue this problem and create adverse effects on the labour market.

Physicians for a National Health Program

Physicians for a National Health Program (PNHP) was founded in 1987 to promote comprehensive health care for all Americans.[2,3] If the Heritage proposal represents the conservative extreme in proposals to reform the US health care system, the PNHP plan represents the liberal extreme.

Underlying goals and values

The stated objectives of the PNHP's proposal are to: (a) minimise financial barriers to appropriate medical care, (b) distribute costs fairly, and (c) contain costs at reasonable levels. Thus the PNHP proposal explicitly accepts the goals of universal access, cost containment and equity in financing health care. The context of the proposal suggests that maintaining quality standards in health care, enhancing physicians' clinical autonomy, and reducing the medical review 'hassle factor' are also seen as appropriate goals for health system reform.

The PNHP proposal seems to reject the concept of economic self-determination for health care providers and consumers. PNHP sees economic competition in the health care sector as inherently wasteful because of high administrative costs and medical review 'hassles'. Using Havighurst's terms, the PNHP wants to substitute the 'professional paradigm' for the 'market paradigm'.[4] PNHP envisages key decisions about health care being made by committees of health experts and community representatives rather than by individual consumers and health providers.

Perception of the problem

In PNHP's view, the current US health care system is failing. PNHP rejects any solution that leaves the private health insurance system intact because PNHP believes that only by reducing administrative costs can access to health care be expanded while expenditures are contained.

Elements of the proposal

The PNHP proposes that the USA establish a national health programme similar to that in Canada. Under the plan, everyone would be fully insured for all medically necessary services, without deductibles or co-insurance. The specific services and procedures covered by the national plan would be determined by panels of experts and community representatives. An expanded programme of technology assessment and cost-effectiveness evaluation would help guide decisions about what services should be covered.

The private health insurance industry would be almost entirely eliminated because insurance coverage that duplicates the public health plan would be proscribed. Since patients could secure health services not covered by the public plan by paying for them directly, a small private insurance industry might continue to exist.

The national health programme would disburse virtually all payments for health services. Each hospital would negotiate with a national health payment board for an annual lump sum payment to cover operating expenses. Funds for facility renovation and expansion and for the purchase of equipment would be distributed by state and regional health-planning boards. Existing proprietary facilities would receive a fair rate of return on existing capital but new for-profit investment would be proscribed.

Facilities such as hospitals, health centres, clinics and group practices could choose to receive a global budget covering a range of services, including physicians' services. Physicians employed in such institutions would be salaried.

Health maintenance organisations (HMO's) and group practices could elect to be paid on a capitation basis for outpatient services, physicians' services and home health care. The capitation fee would not cover hospital inpatient services, except those provided by the HMO physicians. Physicians working in an HMO would be salaried. Physicians could also choose fee-for-service practice. Physician representatives would negotiate a fee schedule with state health plans. This fee schedule would apply to all physicians in fee-for-service practice, and 'balance billing' for services covered by the national health plan would not be permitted. An expenditure cap would be established for physicians' services provided under fee-for-service practice. If spending exceeded the cap, fee levels would be lowered.

Another expert panel would select which drugs and outpatient equipment would be covered by the national plan. Suppliers would bill the national health plan directly for the wholesale cost of the drug or equipment.

PNHP believes that all, or much, of the additional costs of a national health programme can be covered by eliminating 'unnecessary' administrative costs. Bringing the utilisation levels of the uninsured up to the levels of the insured population would cost about $12.2 billion. According to PNHP, this amount could be more than made up by the administrative savings that a single-payer national health plan could achieve. However, PNHP admits that the impact of such a programme on utilisation levels is difficult to predict. Nevertheless, PNHP believes that the monopsony power of government could keep expenditure growth under control.

Trade-offs

In terms of social trade-offs, the PNHP offers strong cost containment, universal access to health care, maintenance of quality standards, and a reduction in administrative hassles. These benefits would be achieved by reducing physicians' economic freedom, reducing freedom of choice for health care consumers, reducing the access of patients to certain types of medical procedures and technologies, and by causing some temporary job dislocation in the health sector.

Feasibility

The feasibility of the PNHP proposal is probably low because it requires massive structural change in the US health care system. Implementation of the proposal would require a large increase in taxes and an expanded role for governments—changes that are likely to be strongly opposed by a significant proportion of the US electorate. Opinion surveys consistently find little public confidence in the ability of governments to run the health care system efficiently.

The feasibility of the proposal is also low because it is likely to be opposed vigorously by health sector organisations. Health insurers would probably lead the opposition to the plan because their businesses would be eliminated or severely reduced. Since private, for-profit investment would be phased out by the plan, the proprietary hospital sector is also likely to oppose the PNHP proposal. Not-for-profit hospitals are not likely to support the PNHP plan because it offers no assurances that the global budgets set for hospitals will be adequate. Physicians are likely to oppose the PNHP plan because of its potential to reduce clinical and economic autonomy and to lead to reductions in physician income levels. The provision that fees will be lowered if the expenditure cap is exceeded would in itself ensure vigorous opposition from physicians.

Comment and summary

The PNHP proposal describes the institutional structure of a single payer system but does not explain how the institutions will interact with each other. For example, committees of experts would determine what would be covered by the national health plan. Exactly how such decisions would be made is unclear. Further, the adjustment process for situations where coverage policy is inconsistent with the politically determined allocation of GDP to health care is not described. No system to ensure that quality standards are maintained is described.

Throughout, the PNHP proposal confuses measured cost with true social cost. For example, the proposal points to Canada as an example of how a single-payer health care system can contain expenditures. Relative to the USA, Canada does spend a smaller percentage of its GDP on health care. But one of the ways that Canada achieves lower measured health care costs is by limiting the availability of certain types of health care procedures, such as open heart surgery. If a dollar value were attributed to delays imposed upon Canadian patients, the social costs of the Canadian health care system would be higher than its measured costs.

One of the more appealing arguments in the PNHP proposal is the claim that administrative costs in the US health care system could be reduced enough to finance health benefits for the approximately 37 million Americans without health insurance coverage. This claim is controversial and cannot be adequately assessed until more studies of administrative costs are completed.

Enthoven and Kronick

The proposal by Alain Enthoven and Richard Kronick represents another variant of reform proposals.[5,6] Unlike others, Enthoven and Kronick see changes in the organisational structure of medical practice as one of the key components of a strategy to enhance the performance of the health care sector.

Underlying goals and values

The Enthoven–Kronick proposal has two main goals: (i) to ensure that almost all individuals have financial protection against the costs of health care services; and (ii) to reduce the rate of growth of health care costs. The context of the discussion by Enthoven and Kronick suggests that they also have goals of improving the level of economic efficiency in the health care sector and increasing equity in the US health care system.

Although Enthoven and Kronick refer to their proposal as a system designed to promote quality, their papers include very little discussion of quality as a separate goal for the health sector. They seem to see quality as a variable and want to ensure that consumers are making optimal trade-offs between quality and price.

Implicit in the Enthoven–Kronick proposal is the view that health care is different from other goods and services, but exactly what is different is never clearly articulated. The authors clearly state that free market forces have a tendency to result in market failure, apparently defined as not achieving society's goals for the health sector.

In spite of their condemnation of free market forces, Enthoven and Kronick endorse economic competition and free choice as the principles upon which the health care system should be based. Their concept is to use governmental legislative power to establish a system of managed competition that will achieve society's health goals.

Perception of the problem

Enthoven and Kronick emphasise four interrelated failings of the current health care system. First, they see the current system as inefficient and wasteful. Related to the problem of economic inefficiency is the second failing—rising health care costs. The problem of rising costs contributes to the third failing of the current system—inadequate financial protection for health care expenses. They criticise the health sector because segments of the population have inadequate health insurance and because the health insurance industry systematically denies coverage to those who need it the most. The final failing relates to the unfairness of the current system. Enthoven and Kronick see the current system of financing health care as unfair because some individuals receive health coverage that is subsidised by the tax system, while others have no health coverage at all.

For Enthoven and Kronick, the financial incentives inherent in fee-for-service medicine are the primary source of the failings of the current health care system. A key element of their proposal is, therefore, encouraging managed care systems which employ alternatives to the fee-for-service payment system.

Elements of the proposal

To solve the access problem, Enthoven and Kronick would require that employers offer health insurance coverage to full-time employees and their dependants. The employer would have to offer a variety of health insurance plans that meet federal standards. State-level public sponsors would offer health plans to those not covered by employer-provided plans.

Regardless of the insurance plan the employee chooses, the employer's required contribution to the cost of the plan would be limited to 80% of the cost of an average plan meeting federal standards. Employers who choose not to provide health insurance benefits to part-time workers would have to pay an additional payroll tax, which would be allocated to the appropriate public sponsor. Self-employed individuals, early retirees, and others not covered by employer-provided health insurance plans would have to pay an additional income tax, which would also be allocated to the appropriate public sponsor.

The public sponsors would be state-level, quasi-public agencies that would contract with health providers and offer health insurance coverage at 20% of the actual cost of the insurance package to those not covered by employer-provided insurance plans, Medicare or Medicaid. Small businesses could arrange health insurance coverage for their employees through the public sponsor for a given percentage of payroll expenses.

The poor would receive additional governmental subsidies to assist in purchasing health insurance coverage through employers or through public sponsors. The elderly would continue to be covered by Medicare and the poor by Medicaid.

Tax policy would be structured such that an employer's contribution to a health benefit plan that exceeds 80% of the average cost of a qualified plan would be reported as income to the employee. This approach would limit the willingness of employees to demand overly generous health benefits from their employers.

The costs of the public health plans would be financed jointly by the federal and state governments. In general, the federal government would finance 50% of the cost of insuring an individual through a public sponsor, with the state picking up 30% and the individual paying the remaining 20%.

Enthoven and Kronick believe that the incentives in their proposal will result in rapid growth in managed care systems. In their view, managed care systems have inherent advantages over other delivery systems. They see managed care systems competing aggressively with each other, with only the plans that deliver high-quality, low-cost care being able to survive. They also believe that, in the long run, large multi-specialty group practice will be the successful model for medical practice and that physicians will be paid by performance-based systems that are somewhere between fee-for-service, resource-based relative values, and salary.

Trade-offs

The proposal by Enthoven and Kronick seems to offer better control of health care prices and expenditures and a higher percentage of USA residents with coverage for health care services. But most middle-class Americans would probably end up with less comprehensive health insurance coverage than they currently have. If managed care systems proliferate as Enthoven and Kronick envision, both patients and physicians may experience a decline in quality standards and in freedom to make individualised clinical decisions.

Feasibility

The feasibility of the Enthoven–Kronick approach is probably high. The concept of requiring employers to provide basic health insurance to employees has been incorporated into a number of other proposals, including the AMA's Health Access America proposal and the HealthAmerica bill, which are described below. Further, economic competition among managed care systems appears likely to be a key element in the Clinton administration's proposal to reform the US health care system.

Physicians are likely to oppose some elements of the Enthoven–Kronick plan. They are likely to object to permitting quality to be a variable. Physicians are also likely to be concerned about growth of managed care systems unless physicians are assured that they will have an appropriate level of clinical autonomy.

The business community, particularly the small business community, may object to the mandate to provide health benefits. Enthoven and Kronick anticipate this objection and propose letting the minimum wage decline to offset the additional business expense of providing health benefits.

Comment and summary

The Enthoven–Kronick proposal is of interest because it emerged early in the current discussion of health system reform and appears to have had a substantial impact on other 'reformers,' including the Clinton administration. This proposal is generally detailed and well presented. However, their discussion of information on medical procedures and technologies and on quality assurance is vague and incomplete.

HealthAmerica: Affordable Health Care for All Americans Act

'HealthAmerica: Affordable Health Care for All Americans' is a comprehensive legislative reform package (S.1227) crafted by the Senate Democratic leadership and introduced in the Congress in June 1991.

Underlying goals and values

The goals of the HealthAmerica reform proposal are explicitly stated: to guarantee access to health care by 'assuring each person a means of payment for care', and to reduce total national health spending.[7] Indeed, access to health care is presented by the bills' sponsors as a '... right for all Americans, not merely a luxury for those who have the economic means to purchase health insurance'.[7] The legislation also endorses improving the quality of health care through such measures as health outcomes research and provision of information to consumers on the 'quality performance' of individual providers.

The value premises underlying HealthAmerica embrace collective responsibility to address the perceived failures in the health care sector. The uninsured population, for example, is viewed as a societal problem caused by such external forces as rising health care costs and business's failure to universally extend health benefits to their workforce. Recommended solutions incorporate the responsibilities of government and employers to ensure that all Americans have access to a certain basic level of health care, as a matter of entitlement.

Perception of the problem

The HealthAmerica reform proposal identifies two problems with the current health care system: financial barriers that limit access to health care by substantial segments of the population (particularly employed, uninsured adults and their dependants), and rapidly rising health care expenditures. The underlying 'crisis' is depicted as high health care costs which threaten the adequacy and affordability of health insurance for employers and individuals. The 'cost crisis' is attributed to such factors as the provision of 'unnecessary' medical care, inappropriate use and reimbursement policies for new and emerging technologies, and the administrative complexities of the current health insurance and financing system.[7]

Elements of the proposal

The HealthAmerica legislation proposes to achieve universal access to health care through an employment-based model that uses a 'play-or-pay' option. Employers would be required to purchase private health insurance for workers and their dependants or contribute a preset percentage of wages to a new government insurance programme called 'AmeriCare'. Employers that choose to provide private insurance must offer, at a minimum, a basic benefits package and pay the majority (generally 80%) of the insurance premium for the worker and his or her family. The 'play-or-pay' strategy would be phased in over several years with tax help for small businesses to assist them in complying with the new requirement.

The Medicare programme for the elderly would remain intact. Medicaid, however, would be dismantled and replaced by the new public programme, AmeriCare. AmeriCare would insure workers whose employers chose to 'pay' and all persons with incomes below the poverty level. AmeriCare's benefits would be the same as private employer-based plans, with the addition of screening, diagnostic and treatment services for low-income children.

As one of its chief cost-containment mechanisms, HealthAmerica would establish a new independent public agency, the 'Federal Health Expenditures Board'. This Board would set annual targets for total national health spending, and convene and oversee negotiations between health care providers and purchasers to develop prices and payment rates. Other key cost-containment provisions of the bill include small market insurance reform, medical liability reform, and standardisation of health insurance claims and data forms used by payers to reduce the administrative complexity of the health care system.

To promote quality of care under the reformed system outlined in HealthAmerica, new state-level public agencies, called 'Quality Improvement Boards', (QIB) would be established. The QIB would review the quality of care provided in the state and implement a data collection process on provider performance for distribution to consumers. The QIB also would have responsibility for adopting medical practice guidelines, or parameters, and certifying providers as 'outstanding' and therefore exempt from the utilisation review practices of third-party payers.

The HealthAmerica legislative reform package would require an estimated $6 billion in new revenue for the first full year of operation following enactment.[8] Major new financing sources to implement the package are not specified by the bill's sponsors.

Trade-offs

The HealthAmerica reform legislation does not explicitly recognise the inherent trade-offs among society's goals of improving access, controlling costs, and maintaining quality in the health care sector. Clearly, the legislation, if enacted, would encourage health care utilisation among the formerly uninsured, a benefit that may improve individual quality of life as well as labour-force productivity. Such expansion of coverage, however, would undoubtedly contribute to the growth in national health spending. Although the legislation contains several cost-containment provisions to offset some of the added costs, enactment would nonetheless require major new national health outlays.

The major potential cost-saving provision, establishment of the Federal Health Expenditures Board, also has some questionable implications and trade-offs. First, there is no compelling reason to believe that the proposed policies and regulations set forth by the Board would inherently achieve a more economically efficient health care system than the market-based interventions proposed by other reform advocates. Second, it is not economically feasible for a single agency to establish prices for all health care services in all sectors and ensure that neither 'too much' nor 'too little' health care is consumed. Thus, by implication, shortages of certain services (both geographically and by specialty) may invariably result, thereby comprising access goals. Similarly, under the expenditure goals, some restraint on access to and reimbursement for expensive new technologies may occur for consumers and providers.

The legislative proposal also fails to acknowledge fully the substantial impact of the 'play-or-pay' system on the labour market and the general economy. For example, requiring employers to provide coverage or pay into a new public programme could raise the effective wage rate for businesses and potentially reduce cash compensation for workers, increase unemployment rates, raise product prices, and threaten the financial viability of some employers.

Feasibility

Under the HealthAmerica proposal, most Americans would retain their private, employment-based insurance coverage; the remaining would be covered under the new public health insurance plan, AmeriCare. By building on the two basic sources of coverage that prevail in the USA, the proposal may be one of the most politically and culturally acceptable routes to health system reform.

However, the new revenue required to finance the proposal remains a substantial drawback, especially in the light of public and political reticence towards tax increases. Moreover, opposition to the proposal in the business community, especially among small firms, is formidable, as many firms continue to oppose any bill that would potentially increase labour costs.

Overall, the acceptance of the proposal by business, as well as its viability in the health system reform discussions, hinges on the legislative approach to cost containment. Yet many of the strategies that would most appeal to employers, such as expenditure targets, will alienate the provider community and threaten consumers' level of access to health care services.

Comment and summary

The HealthAmerica legislative reform package promotes universal access to health care through expanded employer responsibility for coverage and new government policies and programmes. A fundamental concern with the legislation, however, is its apparent acceptance of the belief that increased government regulation and new public agencies can, without provider or consumer incentives, significantly improve the efficiency of the health care sector.

The legislation does contain some market-based incentives to moderate costs and improve efficiency, including: co-insurance and deductible requirements in the mandated minimum benefits plan; insurance market reforms to force insurers to eliminate medical underwriting as a competitive strategy; and encouragement of managed care initiatives in the private and public sector. Nonetheless, the legislation would create new layers of bureaucracy and a central authority to determine health care prices and resource allocation. Such administratively complex pricing mechanisms could lead to implicit rationing through denial of beneficial care and impede technological advancements in the health care sector.

Health Access America

The American Medical Association (AMA) announced its reform proposal, Health Access America, in March of 1990. The comprehensive proposal consists of several key principles and provisions designed to improve access to affordable, high-quality health care.[9]

Underlying goals and values

The stated goals of the AMA reform proposal are to: expand access to health care; control inappropriate rising health care expenditures; foster a continued level of high-quality health care; and ensure individual freedom of choice in selecting the type of insurance coverage and health care they receive. The proposal advocates that these goals can be achieved through selected government intervention and a private-market focus that encourages competition in the health care sector.

Preserving the strengths of the current health care system

(e.g. the widespread availability of employment-based coverage and the accessibility of new technologies for most Americans) is a basic tenet of the AMA proposal. Maintaining the professional independence of practitioners, whereby physicians are able 'to act as patient advocates rather than agents of the government' is also discussed in the proposal as a crucial element of the American health care system that must be preserved and fostered under any reform scenario.[10]

Perception of the problem

The AMA proposal discusses two main problems with the health care system: limited financial access to health care for a substantial proportion of Americans, and rising health care costs. The 'access problem' is viewed as a financing issue caused by inadequacies in the Medicaid programme for the poor and the uncertainty of employment-based coverage for the workforce.

The 'cost problem' is attributed to many factors: new and expensive technology, aggregate population growth, general and medical care price inflation, and the health problems associated with social problems such as violence, drug abuse, poverty, and AIDS. 'Defensive medicine' activities, excessive paperwork and insurance administration, and medical care delivered outside of professionally developed and accepted practice parameters are also viewed as contributing substantially to the overall growth in national health spending.

Elements of the proposal

The AMA proposes to expand access to health care through an employment-based model that would require all firms to provide insurance coverage to their workforce. This insurance must include, at a minimum, coverage for basic health benefits with 'reasonable' annual limits on employees' incurred expenses for premiums, co-insurance, and deductibles. The mandate would be phased in over several years, with tax incentives for employers to help them comply with the new requirement.

Other proposed modifications to the current system of employer-sponsored health insurance include: pre-empting state-mandated health benefit laws to help small businesses afford basic coverage for their workers; ending the current exemption of self-insured employers from participation in such health insurance coverage requirements as state risk pools, and eliminating provisions that exclude pre-existing conditions from employer health benefit plans.

The Medicaid programme would remain intact under the AMA proposal, although eligibility criteria would be modified. Current categorical standards would be replaced with a national formula, so that Medicaid would cover all individuals with incomes below 100% of the poverty level. Medicaid's benefits would be standardised with a national, uniform floor of coverage for physician, hospital and other services. These changes would be phased in over several years, with an initial focus on expanding coverage for all pregnant women and children below the poverty level.

Additionally, the AMA proposal recommends reforming government financing of the Medicare programme. An enhanced Medicare trust fund would be established and funded beyond immediate payout needs (refunding) through individual and employer tax contributions during the working years. Long-term care coverage for the elderly would also be expanded by creating tax incentives for the purchase of private sector coverage.

The AMA approach to cost containment emphasises market-based strategies to encourage competition and informed consumer decision-making. Health care providers, for example, would be required to release fees for frequently provided services to consumers before treatment. Cost containment would also be encouraged by altering individual incentives to 'over-insure'. The tax treatment of employer-provided benefits would be changed to remove the existing regressive subsidisation of health care benefits and government rebates offered to employees who select 'economical' insurance plans from their employer. Other cost-containment measures advocated by the AMA include: reforming the small group health insurance market to improve the affordability and availability of private coverage; reducing the administrative costs of health care by requiring all private insurers to use standard claim forms; pursuing professional liability reform to reduce the inappropriate costs of defensive medicine and liability insurance premiums; and enacting legislation to allow medical societies to review patient complaints about physicians' fees and to mediate voluntary agreements between patients and physicians.

The AMA plan proposes to enhance the quality of health care services through practice parameters and legislative initiatives to assure adequate funding for health care outcomes research. Other quality-related initiatives include expanded federal support for medical education and intensified health promotion and disease prevention programmes.

Trade-offs

The AMA proposal explicitly acknowledges the inherent trade-offs among society's goals of access, cost and quality for the health care sector. Throughout, the AMA notes that expanding access to care for the uninsured cannot be achieved without additional health care expenditures. However, the AMA believes that this goal merits additional resources; whether the general public, Congress, and the current Administration agree with this assessment is questionable.

Mandated employer-sponsored insurance, the cornerstone of the AMA's proposal to expand access, would also add a fixed sum to the cost of labour that is not explicitly acknowledged in the reform proposal. Standard economic analysis suggests that the cost of this insurance eventually will be reflected in lower wages or higher product prices than otherwise would have occurred in the absence of the mandate. Although the proposal includes tax incentives to new and small employers, these incentives may not completely offset the potentially deleterious effects on business and the labour market.

Feasibility

The AMA reform proposal represents a relatively comprehensive approach to expanding access and attempts to address the issue of rising health care costs through market-based forces that encourage competition in the health care economy. However, the access elements form the proposal's strongest plank. Compared to other competing reform proposals, the AMA's cost-containment provisions lack the explicit budgetary controls or economic incentives to encourage efficiency in the health care market. The overall questionable impact of the AMA proposal on national health spending, coupled with the estimated $21 billion cost to the federal government of implementing the proposal, may hinder its political feasibility in the current era of fiscal constraint.[10]

The AMA reform proposal also does not involve significant deviation from a competitive market for health care services or insurance. Neither physicians nor insurers are likely to object to most of the proposal's features. However, the employer mandates could arouse opposition from the business community despite the tax incentives offered to help offset the cost of such coverage. This opposition and the proposal's relatively high price tag for the federal coffers may forestall the otherwise formidable gains in insurance coverage and health care access that could be achieved through implementation of the AMA proposal.

Comment and summary

On the continuum of health care reform plans, the AMA proposal falls in the middle ground, emphasising competitive forces and other market-driven solutions to the cost issue while promoting some government-based intervention to extend access to care. The proposal is generally non-intrusive with respect to providers and payers of health care, and provides several mechanisms to promote near-universal coverage to a basic level of health services through the existing bureaucracy.

The proposal also retains a decentralised, competitive private health insurance market with new incentives to encourage cost-sharing and consumer cost consciousness in the private sector. However, like all market-based solutions, the AMA proposal cannot offer any guarantees on the ultimate aggregate level of health expenditures following its implementation.

CHOICES IN HEALTH SYSTEM REFORM

Although only five of the more than 50 proposals to reform the US health care system are reviewed in this chapter, those five are indicative of the types of strategies currently being considered under the rubric of reforming the US health sector. They also illustrate the difficult trade-offs that may have to be made among health goals. Drawing primarily on the analyses of the five proposals presented above, this section provides a general overview of the choice set that seems to have been established by the current debate over how to reform the US health care system.

Access

The most distinctive difference among health system reform proposals is in the methods that they would use to improve access (widely defined as increasing the percentage of the population covered by adequate health insurance or benefit plans). Three alternative approaches are advocated: (i) requiring individuals and families to purchase health benefit packages; (ii) mandating that employers provide health benefit coverage to employees and their families; and (iii) establishing a national health plan in which governments provide health benefit coverage to all citizens. A fourth approach, proposed by former President Bush, would use tax policy to encourage individuals and businesses to purchase private health insurance voluntarily. In discussions of health system reform, these four alternatives often serve as a classification system because

Table 9.1 Improving access: strategies and mechanisms

Strategies	Mechanisms
Voluntary approach: give individuals/ business incentives to purchase health insurance	• Use legislation to reform the small group insurance market (establish community rating), encourage development of business groups to negotiate with private insurers, and provide additional tax deductions/credits to subsidise purchase of private health insurance.[11] (Bush Administration)
Individual mandate: require households to purchase health insurance	• Enact legislation to require households to purchase health insurance and use tax credits and deductions to help households purchase private health insurance (Heritage)
Employer mandate (two major variations)	• Employer required to provide basic coverage for all full-time employees and their families (the play-all-the-way option) — part-time workers given vouchers to purchase private insurance and state risk pools established (AMA) — additional payroll tax imposed to fund coverage for part-time workers through public sponsors. (Enthoven and Kronick)
	• Employer provides basic coverage for all employees and families or pays additional payroll tax (the play-or-pay option). New public plan established for those not covered through employment setting or Medicare (HealthAmerica)
National health insurance (two major used variations)	• Establish new plan in which administrative mechanisms (rather than market mechanisms) are used to make key decisions and allocate health resources (PNHP) • Extend existing federal Medicare system, with its limited incentives for consumers to economise, to all age categories[12]

a proposal can be based on only one of them. Table 9.1 outlines the four alternatives and their major implementation mechanisms.

Cost

Three basic strategies to contain health care expenditures are advocated in proposals to reform the US health care system: (i) reduce or stabilise health care prices and fees; (ii) reduce or stabilise utilisation of health care; and (iii) control health care expenditures directly. The mechanisms to reduce prices and fees are outlined in Table 9.2 and those designed to reduce utilisation are presented in Table 9.3. In contrast to the mechanisms proposed to improve access, the mechanisms to contain health care costs are frequently complementary approaches, rather than distinct alternatives.

The third strategy—directly controlling health care expenditures—is more of a concept than a proposal. Although the Clinton administration has promoted the idea of 'global budgets' for health care, the method to enforce a limit on health spending has not yet been articulated. The PNHP proposal recommends reducing physicians' fees in a future year if the spending cap is exceeded in a given year. The idea seems to be that the supply of physicians' services is highly inelastic and that current fee levels include considerable economic rent and, consequently, fees can be driven down without affecting supply in a significant way. The risk of such an enforcement system is that some prices could be driven below their corresponding marginal costs, reducing the availability of some services.

Several US Congressmen have begun to look at the German system, in which fees and expenditures on physicians' services are negotiated at the beginning of the year. If the expenditure target is exceeded, the fees that physicians actually receive are lower than the negotiated rates. Thus far, this approach has not been incorporated into any proposals to reform the US health care system.

Table 9.2 Controlling health care costs: price/expenditures strategies and mechanisms

Strategies	Mechanisms
Enhance price competition	• Make price/fee information readily available to potential customers (AMA) • Use tax policy to encourage higher co-insurance rates and deductibles, thereby giving consumers stronger incentives to search (Heritage, AMA) • Encourage large group practices that aggressively compete with each other (Enthoven and Kronick) • Establish fee review committees to mediate fee disputes (AMA)
Reduce production costs	• Reduce administrative costs by standardising billing, record keeping, etc. (AMA, PNHP) • Enact professional liability reform to reduce cost of liability insurance (AMA) • Reduce excess capacity through regulation of capital equipment and facilities (used by many state governments) • Use monopsony power of government to drive down prices of inputs such as drugs and medical equipment (PNHP)
Directly control prices	• Negotiate or regulate fees and prices of medical services (PNHP)
Fee discounts for the poor	• Encourage charity care (AMA) • Limit 'balance billing' to poor patients (AMA)

Table 9.3 Controlling costs: utilisation strategies and mechanisms

Strategies	Mechanisms
Reduce demand	• Using tax policy, encourage higher co-insurance rates and deductibles (Heritage, AMA) • Use variable co-insurance rates to reflect social prioritisation of types of health care services (State of Oregon) • Encourage managed care techniques such as second opinion and prior authorisation (widely used in USA) • Through variable co-insurance rates, encourage patients to access specialists through a primary care physician—the gatekeeper approach[13] (American Academy of Family Practice) • Encourage healthy lifestyles and preventive care (AMA)
Reduce health problems	• Reduce social/public health environmental problems that generate need for health care services (AMA)
Change physician behaviour	• Promote prepaid group practice (Enthoven and Kronick) • Reduce risk of professional liability claims (AMA) • Develop/distribute practice parameters (AMA, HealthAmerica) • Develop effective peer/medical review (AMA)
Control diffusion of new medical technologies	• Establish evaluation commission (PNHP)

Quality

Quality receives little attention in the current set of reform proposals, except those developed by provider groups. Almost no discussion exists on how medical review should be conducted to ensure that the patient actually receives the quality of care that is being paid for. Most proposals implicitly recognise that poor-quality care can exacerbate the health care cost problem by forcing patients to repeat medical treatments. Most of the discussion of effectiveness research is in terms of cost containment rather than quality enhancement. The focus is primarily on eliminating ineffective procedures and encouraging more economically efficient ways to deliver existing medical technologies.

Proposed mechanisms to improve quality include: developing and distributing practice parameters to physicians, increasing funding for outcomes research, and increasing the funding for medical research. Several proposals recommend the establishment of national or regional quality boards to oversee the implementation of these mechanisms.

Trade-offs

Implicit in the current set of reform proposals are a variety of choices for trade-offs among the goals of cost, quality and access. Most proposals would reduce the typical American's level of access (defined as potential command over health care resources) in order to achieve cost containment and universal access (defined as every American being covered by at least a basic health insurance or health benefit plan). Extending basic health benefits to all Americans will tend to increase health care expenditures. To offset this effect, many reform proposals would reduce the services covered by existing, 'overly generous' health benefit plans and would increase deductibles and co-insurance rates for most Americans already covered by health plans. In general, the reform proposals that advocate a single national plan (similar to the Canadian model) offer strict cost containment, universal access (everyone has a health benefit plan), and maintenance of quality standards for procedures, by: reducing the clinical and economic autonomy of health providers; increasing tax rates and the role of governments in the health sector; reducing the health care choices available to patients; possibly reducing medical innovation; and possibly increasing waiting times for certain types of care. Although individuals would have little or no out-of-pocket expenses for covered care, the ability of individual patients and physicians to select certain types of care would be limited by regulatory mechanisms. Other regulatory mechanisms would probably ensure that the quality of health care services delivered would continue to be adequate, but the perceived overall quality of the health care system could decline if individual choice is severely curtailed and if long waiting periods for non-emergency care occur. Inadequate supplies of health personnel could occur in the long run if controls on fees and incomes make the health professions less attractive career choices.

Generalising about the employer mandate proposals is difficult because many variations exist. The play-or-pay variations would help contain health care expenses by increasing the role of the federal government in the health sector and by reducing the economic autonomy of providers. A frequently expressed concern about the play-or-pay variation is that the parameters of the system could be manipulated in a way that employers increasingly choose the 'pay option' and the system evolves *de facto* into a national health insurance plan.

The reform proposals that would require households to purchase private health insurance seem to offer universal access, strict cost containment, and a reduction in the direct role of government in the health care sector, by: significantly reducing the typical individual's potential command over health care resources; increasing taxes; and by possibly permitting quality standards to decline. The proposals that would encourage voluntary purchases of private health insurance seem to offer improved access and maintenance of quality standards by trading off higher taxes and health expenditures.

Increasing the level of economic efficiency in the health sector is often seen as a way to avoid the inherent trade-off among other goals. The typical argument is that health care prices and expenditures could be reduced without adversely affecting quality and access if the health sector could be induced to produce with the least cost combination of resources, and if unnecessary or low benefit care could be reduced or eliminated. Reform proposals almost never discuss the effects on economic efficiency that occur because health insurance creates a wedge between the price of the health care product, as seen by the consumer, and the social cost of that product. But the trade-off among goals cannot be completely avoided. At some point, achieving further increases in economic efficiency may require increasing co-insurance rates to give patients stronger incentives to seek cost-effective care, but that policy implies some decrease in access.

Similarities

Although the current set of reform proposals are different in many ways, they also have many points of similarity. For example, they would all use legislation to modify the structure of the US health care sector in order to change its economic performance. Another similarity is that the major reform proposals (with the possible exception of the Heritage proposal) explicitly or implicitly endorse the view that the health care product is somewhat unique and that society's goals for the health sector differ from those of other sectors. Consequently, none of the proposals argue that laissez-faire economic competition is the appropriate economic paradigm for the health care sector.

The current set of reform proposals are also similar in the factors that are not targeted for change. With the exception of encouraging the growth of prepaid group practice, most proposals do not advocate changing the existing approach to producing health care. The medical roles and relationships among physicians, hospitals and other medical professionals are left unchanged. None of the proposals would change the legal infrastructure, such as the state-level medical practice acts, that set the basic parameters within which medical care is produced and delivered. None of the proposals explicitly advocates permitting the quality of medical care to vary more widely in order to give health care consumers more choice (possibly a desirable social goal in itself) and, thereby, increase the level of price competition in the health care sector. None of the proposals would institute explicit non-market rationing of health care services; individual patients would not be proscribed from consuming particular services because of their demographic or medical characteristics. Changing the content of medical education as a mechanism to influence the economic performance of the health sector is given very little attention in the proposals. Further, issues relating to the role of society in subsidising the educational costs of health professionals, supply and geographic distribution of health resources, the level and focus of medical research, and the diffusion of medical advances are usually not discussed in any detail. Somewhat surprising is the limited recognition that advances in medical technology can be a way to avoid the difficult trade-offs among the health goals of cost, quality and access. Advances in medical technology are usually seen as increasing health care prices and expenditures. But history suggests that medical innovations (e.g. the treatment of tuberculosis with antibiotics) can also lead to reductions in expenditures and to higher-quality medical outcomes. Also surprising is the limited recognition that social problems (violence, drugs, environmental pollution) and unhealthy lifestyles contribute to the problem of high and rising health care expenditures.

POLITICS OF HEALTH SYSTEM REFORM

Virtually all economic and political interest groups in the USA agree that major reform of the health care system is necessary and that the American public wants some kind of reform to take place.[14] However, two factors have prevented the coalescence of political will necessary to achieve reform. One factor is disagreements among political and economic interest groups about what kind of reform should be implemented[15]—the nature of these disagreements is evident from the differences in the health care reform proposals discussed earlier in this chapter. The second and more important factor is money. Any one of the health care reform proposals, no matter where it sits on the ideological spectrum, is likely to result in large increases in spending on health care. The increases would occur because all of the proposals would finance health care for the millions of people who are uninsured and underinsured; and large amounts of money would have to be found for this coverage. The measures that would have to be implemented to prevent health expenditures from rising are Draconian and would be vigorously opposed by health providers and others.

Although the American public wants health care reform, the majority have not demonstrated the will to support the additional expenditures. To finance health system reform, steps might include: increasing taxes (directly or indirectly); eliminating other government programmes; or increasing the debt levels of the federal government and state governments. These are courses of action that the American public has clearly rejected and, therefore, no politician wants to be accountable for pursuing them. The public desire for reform coupled with the lack of will to make the necessary sacrifices is a serious dilemma for governments. The political battles necessary to settle the ideological differences about reform would probably have been fought and resolved by now if the financing problem was not so acute.

Because of the financial problem, a comprehensive health care reform bill is unlikely to be passed at the federal or state level in the near future. Instead, incremental health reform legislation will probably be enacted. Such legislation will impose mechanisms such as price controls on hospitals and physicians in the private sector, or measures designed to increase the amount of competition for managed care contracts, but will not fundamentally alter the health care system. It will also marginally expand the number of uninsured individuals eligible for government health plans, but will not provide universal access to care. More dramatic reform will be deferred by authorising the creation of government commissions to make studies and recommendations about what further reforms should be implemented. These commissions or other entities may be designed in a way that permits them to evolve into the bureaucratic structure necessary to manage a new health reform system.

This course of action will allow governments to demonstrate that some action has been taken to resolve the problems of cost and access without committing to spend the additional money needed to cover all of the uninsured and underinsured. Measures such as price controls on hospitals and physicians are likely to be very popular with the public and to take some pressure off governments to do more on health system reform. The states of Florida,[16] Minnesota,[17] and Vermont[18] have already passed incremental legislation, and similar bills are pending in many other states.[19]

After incremental reforms have been implemented, pressure will continue to build for more comprehensive reforms. Advocates for the uninsured and the underinsured will continue lobbying to extend coverage to those populations. Although price controls may provide some temporary relief from price and expenditure increases, experience in the Medicare programme indicates that expenditures will continue to rise, and that providers will become increasingly contentious as the government reacts by further limiting price increases. Private sector payers, especially employers, will continue to seek ways to reduce their health outlays. Most private payers will experiment with managed care and, if that fails to result in significant savings, they will reduce or eliminate employee health care benefits. As the ranks of the uninsured and underinsured increase, and as more members of the public perceive that they might lose coverage, the pressure for more comprehensive reforms will grow. Enough concern may eventually develop over access to health care to generate support for the financial sacrifices necessary to support fundamental health care reform.

Predicting the type of health system reform that might be implemented as a result of this process is difficult. A strong possibility is that the system will evolve from the structure put in place by incremental reform legislation. If the Democratic Party continues to dominate that process, the system that will evolve will likely stress centralised government regulation or outright control of the system. However, if the Republicans regain control of the process of enacting incremental reforms, the future health care system will emphasise economic competition and individual responsibility.

REFERENCES

1. Butler, S. and Haislmaier, E. *A National Health System for America*, Washington, DC, Heritage Foundation, 1989.
2. Himmelstein, D. and Woolhandler, S. A national health program for the United States: a physicians' proposal. *New England Journal of Medicine* 1989; **320**: 102–108.
3. Grumbach, K., Bodenheimer, T., Himmelstein, D. and Woolhandler, S. Liberal benefits, conservative spending: the Physicians for a National Health Program proposal. *Journal of the American Medical Association* 1991; **265**: 2549–2554.
4. Havighurst, C. Michael M. Davis Lecture: The Antitrust Challenge to the Professional Paradigm of Medical Care. In: *Antitrust Intervention in the Health Care Industry*, Proceedings of the Thirty-second Annual George Bugbee Symposium on Hospital Affairs. Chicago: CHAS Publications, Graduate School of Business, University of Chicago, 1990.
5. Enthoven, A. and Kronick, R. A consumer-choice health plan for the 1990s: universal health insurance in a system designed to promote quality and economy. *New England Journal of Medicine* 1989; **320**: 29–37, 92–101.
6. Enthoven, A. and Kronick, R. Universal health insurance through incentives reform. *Journal of the American Medical Association* 1991; **265**: 2532–2536.
7. Mitchell, G. (Democrat, Maine). HealthAmerica: Affordable Health Care For All Americans Act. *Congressional Record* June 5, 1991; **137**: S7175–S7221.
8. American Association of Retired Persons. Confused about health care reform plans? *AARP Bulletin* 1992; **33(1)**: 12.

9. *Health Access America: The AMA Plan to Reform America's Health Care System*. Chicago: American Medical Association, 1992.
10. Todd, J., Seekins, S., Krichbaum, J. and Harvey, L. Health access America: strengthening the US health care system. *Journal of the American Medical Association* 1991; **265**: 2503–2506.
11. *The President's Comprehensive Health Reform Program*. Washington, DC, Government Printing Office, 1992.
12. Davis, K. Expanding Medicare and employer plans to achieve universal health insurance. *Journal of the American Medical Association* 1991; **265**: 2525–2528.
13. *Rx for Health: the Family Physicians' Access Plan*, Kansas City, American Academy of Family Physicians, 1992.
14. Beardsley, T. Better care, less care: can rationing cure the ailing US health care system? *Scientific American* 1992; **266(5)**: 17–20.
15. Noble, L. Healthcare reform stews in congressional pressure cooker. *Healthcare Financial Management* January 1992: 21–39.
16. The New Agency for Health Care Administration and Health Care Reform Act of 1992, Florida Senate Bill No. 2390, 1992 Session.
17. Minnesota House File No. 2800, 2nd year, 77th Session.
18. An Act Relating to a Health Care Authority, Vermont House Bill 733, 1992 Session.
19. Thompson, R. Prescriptions for medical costs. *Nation's Business* 1991; **79(9)**: 38–39.

Index

Access to health care. *See* Health care access
Accreditation process 122
Acute care 92–3
Administrative costs 78–9, 82
Administrative percentage 77
Administrative waste 76
Advisory Committee on Health Manpower 158
Agency relationship 19
Agency utility maximisation model 181–2
AIDS 81, 204, 217, 257
Allocation of services 50
Ambulatory care, quality assurance 125
American College of Physicians 25
American Medical Association (AMA) 26, 53, 251, 256–61
AmeriCare 253
Antibiotics 117
Arthritis 16
Aspirin 16
Audit programmes 122–3, 126, 157
Autonomy of patient 19

Benefit
  measures of 11
  notion of 22
  see also Cost-benefit issues
Black Report 55
Blue Cross 28, 32, 38, 71, 81, 212
Blue Shield 212
Budgetary performance 184
Budgets 16, 17, 46–7, 86
  allocation 112
  capital 144
  management 185, 186

Caesarian section 124
Canada Health Act 1984 31, 57, 113, 114
Canadian health care system 25–66
  annual surgical rates 40
  changing position of organised medicine 51–3
  chronicity issue 162
  community-based approaches 163
  comparison with USA 58, 85
  cost containment 41
  current administrative features 32–5
  evolution to universality 28–32
  expenditure 35–42
  fiscal federalism 56–7
  funding 32–3, 142–5
  future directions 58–9
  health care delivery initiatives 44–7
  health care rationing 48–50

Canadian health care system (*cont.*)
  hospital admissions 40
  hospital bed-days 41
  hospital occupancy rates 35
  hospital sector cost differences 39–42
  hospital services 34–5
  human resources management 141–68
  long-term care 94–5
  management methods 44–7
  medical manpower growth 42–4
  misallocation of resources 52
  per capita claim rate 42
  physicians' earnings 33, 42
  planning approach 163
  population–physician ratio 41
  pressures within 162
  quality assurance 111–39
  services *vs*. pensions 104–7
  surveys of users 53
Canadian Hospital Association 57
Canadian Medical Association 153
Canadian Post-MD Education Registry 151
Canadian Task Fource on the Periodic Health Examination 47
Cancer survival 19
Capital budgets 144
Carotid endarterectomies 117
Case-mix adjustments 47
Case-mix reimbursement systems 102
Case study 4
Cataract surgery 49
Charter of Rights and Freedoms 44
Clinical guidelines 51
Clinical judgement 50
Colleges of Physicians and Surgeons 157
Collegial controls 51
Communication skills, asymmetry in 20
Community advisory councils 119
Community-based care services 92, 98, 103–4
  Canada 163
  funding for 175–7
  health centres 52
  quality assurance 175–7
  regulatory impetus 174–5
  residential 169–95
Community rating 84
Competition model 233
Complaints investigations 127
Compliance 18–19
Comprehensive health organisations 46
Comprehensive Services and Developmental Disabilities Amendments 174
Compulsory payments 74
Conference of Federal, Provincial and Territorial Deputy Ministers of Health 165
Consumer demand 205
Consumer participation 114
  in medical decision-making 52
  in quality of care 119
Consumer Price Index (CPI) 201–2

Continuing education 127
Continuous quality improvement (CQI) 128–30, 132
Coronary angiography 50, 117
Coronary bypass surgery 99
Coronary revascularisation 49
Cost 9–11
Cost-benefit issues 8, 9, 17, 18, 21
Cost-cutting measures 117
Cost-effectiveness 6, 14, 120, 163
Cost-quality-access goals 230
Cost-quality trade-off 169–95, 173
Cost savings-quality trade-off 169–95
Current Population Survey (CPS) 213–14

Data collection, quality assurance 125–6
Decision-making
  economics in 10–11
  macro level of 10
  resource allocation 7–8
Defensive medicine 200, 205
Delay *vs.* denial 48
Demographic influences 204
Dental care programme 157
Dentists 146–7
Department of National Health and Welfare 158
Developmental Disabilities Act 1970 174
Developmental Disabilities Act 1984 174
Developmental Disabilities Assistance Act 1975 174
Developmentally disabled persons
  long-term care 170–8
  residential services 171–8
Diabetes 217
Disabled persons 104
Doctor–patient relationship 14–20, 29
  asymmetry in 19
Doctor–population ratio 44
Drinking 83
Drug cap 117
Drug co-payments 117
Drug costs 144
Drug expenditure 144
'Dumping' phenomenon 49

Economic considerations 9
  in decision-making 10–11
Economic perspective and efficiency 208
Effectiveness 4, 5–6
  evaluation of 235
Efficacy 4
Efficiency 3–9, 21–2
  and economic perpective 208
  and equity 14
  definitions 3–9
  morality of 3–9
Employer perspective 207
Enthoven–Kronick proposal 247–51
  elements of 249–50
  feasibility of 250–1
  goals and values 247–8
  perception of problem 248–9
  trade-offs 250
Equalisation payments 57
Equitable allocation and resource allocation 14

Equity 2, 22, 54, 68–74, 80, 86–7
and efficiency 14
and need 11–14
bottom-up *vs.* top-down 73–4, 86–8
Established Programs Financing (EPF) Act 1977 142
Ethical issues 2, 7, 9, 10, 70, 233
Ethics, President's Commission on 72
Exercising 83

Fairness
in health care services 70–2, 79–85
in medical care 69
to providers 85–6
Federal Health Expenditures Board 253, 254
Federal–Provincial–Territorial Advisory Committee on Health Manpower 159
Fiscal federalism 56–7
Funding
Canadian health care system 32–3, 142–5
community-based programmes 175–7
human resources 142–5
long-term care services for the developmentally disabled 170

General practice
comparison of USA and Canada 85
distribution of services 156
Genetic diseases 84
Geriatric centres 102
Geriatric evaluation units 99
Global budgetary system 46
Government intervention 234
Government perspective 206
Great Depression 28
Greater Victoria Hospital Society 45
Gross domestic product (GDP) 200, 227–8, 247, 263
Gross national product (GNP) 30, 35–6, 38, 41, 56, 68, 75, 91, 112, 142, 143, 198, 199
Guaranteed renewability 84
Gynaecology 43

Handicapped and Disabilities Act 1991 174
Hawaii, single-tap theory 38
Health Access America 256–61
elements of proposal 257–9
feasibility of 260
goals and values 256–7
perception of problem 257
proposal 251
trade-offs 259
Health care access 2, 209–18, 257
components of 229
in reform proposals 261–3
Health care costs 163, 199–208, 257
administrative 78–9, 82
containment 41, 78–9
control 115
in doctor–patient relationship 14–15
increases 198

medical services 71
price/expenditures strategies and mechanisms 264
taxation 74–9
utilisation strategies and mechanisms 265
see also Cost
Health care delivery initiatives 44–7
Health care expenditure 112, 142–3
as percentage of GNP 112, 143
Canadian–American comparisons 35–42
causes of rising 200–5
comparisons of 37
differentials as percentage of GNP 39
international comparisons 199–200
reform proposals 263–5
trends in 199–200, 205–6
Health Care Financing Administration (HCFA) 172
Health care management methods 44–7
Health care professionals
governance practice 156–7
Health care providers
autonomy 50
fairness to 85–6
reactions to reforms 237–8
satisfaction 53–4
Health care rationing
Canada 48–50
USA 48–50
Health care services
limitations 115
objective 3
performance indicators 55
role and importance of 115
Health care system reform
access improvement strategies and mechanisms 261–3
broad questions concerning 226–7
choices in 261–9
definition 225–38
effects on key components of health sector 235–6
failures of current system 231–2
framework for analysis 225–38
goals of 227–31
paradigms and values providing foundation for 232–4
political feasibility assessment 237–8
politics of 269–72
proposals 197–273
public attitudinal surveys 238
quality assurance 266
questions concerning 234
reactions of providers and interest groups 237
review and analysis of major proposals 238–61
similarities in 268–9
social trade-offs 236–7
trade-offs 266–8
see also under specific proposals
Health centres 52
Health insurance 26, 52, 71, 79, 122, 202–3
employment-based 209–10

Health insurance (*cont.*)
  major sources of 209–12
  non-group (or
    self-purchased) 212
  risk-related premiums 81–3
  see also Malpractice; Private
    health insurance;
    Uninsured persons
Health maintenance
    organisations (HMOs) 46,
    71, 81, 245
Health professions 145–56
  self-regulating 157
Health status 115–16, 120
HealthAmerica: Affordable
    Health Care for All
    Americans 251–6
HealthAmerica reform proposal
  elements of 253–4
  feasibility of 255
  goals and values 252
  perception of problem 252
  trade-offs 254–5
Heart disease 217
Heart surgery 49
Heritage foundation
    proposal 238–43
  elements of 240–1
  feasibility of 242
  perception of
    problem 239–40
  trade-offs 241–2
  underlying goals and
    values 238–9
Hill–Burton Act 226
Hip replacement surgery 49
Home care programme
    expenditures 144
Horizontal equity 2
Hospital Medical Records
    Institute (HMRI) 122
Hospitals
  closures 115
  expenditures for 144
  quality assurance 122
  see also Canadian health care
    system
Human resources
  funding 142–5
  health professions 145–56
  management of 141–68
  planning
    approaches 158–60, 163

Individualism 27
Infant mortality 55
Infectious disease 5
Inflation 30–1
Institutional care 92, 98,
    103–4
Insurance. *See* Health
    insurance; Malpractice;
    Private health insurance
Intermediate care facilities for
    the mentally retarded
    (ICF/MR) 170, 176–7
Intra-ocular lens
    replacement 99

Kaiser Permanente 38

Laryngectomy 19
Legislation 119, 226
Libertarianism 27
Licence suspension or
    revocation 127
Life expectancy 54–5, 162,
    200
Lithotripsy 96
Litigation rates 119
Lodge practice 28

Long-term care (LTC) 91–109
  alternative approaches 104
  Canada 94–5
  community-based 101, 169–95
    vs. institutional care 98, 103–4
  concept of 92–3
  decentralisation 102
  developmentally disabled persons 170–8
  endogenous quality model 178–86
  family role in 104
  feasibility issues 95–7, 103–4
  funding 170
  informal support system 93
  institutional *vs.* community-based 98, 103–4
  lessons to be drawn from Canadian experience 103–4
  management of 98–9
  Manitoba model 97, 99–100
  models of 97–103
  Pennsylvania 177–8
  policy questions 92
  previous studies 172–3
  primary care provision 99
  problems of 97
  public support 93
  quality assurance 172, 178–86
  services *vs.* pensions 104–7
  sponsored by social agencies 93
  universal entitlement 96

Macro decisions 11
Macro efficiency/equity judgement 17
Malpractice insurance premiums 42, 205
Manpower growth 42–4
Manpower policy analysis 44
Market forces 234
Medicaid 27, 35, 73, 95, 211–12, 217, 226, 253, 257, 258
Medical Care Act 1968 141, 157
Medical education 166
Medical Illness Severity Grouping System (Medisgroups) 45
Medical insurance. *See* Health insurance
Medical schools 166
  enrolment 159
Medical signature 4
Medicare 26, 29–31, 35, 42, 46, 54, 56, 58, 76, 78, 114, 117, 176, 204, 210–11, 226, 240, 253, 258
  hospital insurance 211
  supplementary medical insurance 211
Medicare Catastrophic Act 1988 211
Mentally retarded persons, intermediate care facilities for (ICF/MR) 170
Minimum coverage 87
Moral hazard 82
Morality of efficiency 3–9

National Committee on Physician Manpower 158
National Demonstration Project 118, 129, 132
National health insurance (NHI) 25, 27, 53, 55, 224

National Health Service 48
Need and equity 11–14
Non-price-rationing 49
Non-steroidal anti-inflammatory drugs (NSAIDs) 16
Nurse–population ratio 148
Nurse-practitioners 44
Nurses and nursing assistants 148–50
Nursing homes 92, 93

Objective of health services 3
Obstetrics 43
Occupational therapists 147–8
Office of Continuing Care 97
Ontario Medical Association (OMA) 45
Open-heart surgery 49, 96
Outcome measurement 7–8

Paediatrics 43
Paramedical personnel 43
Patient
  autonomy of 19
  doctor's responsibility to 20
  see also Doctor–patient relationship
Penalties 127
Pennhurst State Hospital 172
Pennsylvania Office of Mental Retardation 171–2
Pensions *vs.* services 104–7
Pharmacists 145–6
Physician–population ratio 154, 159, 166
Physicians
  activity profile 153
  average gross earnings 42
  distribution of 154–6
  fees for service 164
  future requirements for 159
  immigrants and emigrants 152
  maldistribution of 155
  net income 85
  oversupply problem 159
  referral 99
  remuneration methods 164
  resource planning 159–60, 164
  service expenditures 144
  supply position 150–6
Physicians for a National Health Program (PNHP) 243–7, 263
  elements of proposal 244–5
  feasibility of 246
  goals and values 243–4
  perception of problem 244
  trade-offs 245–6
Physiotherapists 147–8
Political context 26–8, 237–8, 269–72
Population statistics 204
Practice patterns
  assessment of 47
  variations in 116
Practitioner autonomy 52
Practitioner behaviour, techniques employed to influence 127
Prepayment arrangements 52
President's Commission on Ethics 72
Price inflation 201–2
Price rationing 48–9
Principal-agent theory 14
Private health insurance 32, 52, 53, 84, 86, 202, 212, 237–8
Private practice 33, 42, 69, 122

Providers. *See* Health care
providers
Public Hospitals Act 118–19
Public insurance 122

QALY (quality-adjusted life-year) 6–8, 11, 13
Quality assurance 111–39
ambulatory care 125
approaches to 121–7
Canadian health care system 111–39
community-based programmes 175–7
components of 121
consumer participation 119
data collection 125–6
definition 121, 228–9
economic context 112–15
effect of user fees and utilisation caps 117
empirical measures and data 183–4
framework for 123
goals of programming 131–3
health care system reform 266
health impact of poor-quality care 118
hospitals 122
long-term care 172, 178–86
measurement 228–9
operational model 184–6
pre-conditions for 120–1
reform proposals 266
self-regulating health professions 122
shifting focus of 127–31
taxonomy of 178–81
testable hypotheses 184–6
Quality Improvement Boards (QIB) 253
Quality management initiatives 51
Quality-of-life improving 6
Queueing 162
for specialised services 50
in emergency departments 49

Radiation therapy 96
RAND Corporation 117
Rehabilitation Act 1973 174
Rehabilitation Act 1978 174
Reimbursement systems 163
Remuneration methods 166
Requirements Committee 158
Residential services
community-based 169–95
developmentally disabled persons 171–8
Resource allocation 17
and equitable allocation 14
decision-making 7–8
Resource intensity weights 47
Reward system 2
Right to health care 2
Risk-averse persons 81–2
Risk rating 80, 82–4
Risk-related premiums 81–3
Royal Commission on Health Services 158, 164

Scarlet fever 4
Smoking 83
Social problems 257
Social Security 78
Social trade-offs in health care system reform 236–7
Society of Obstetricians and Gynaecologists 124

Socioeconomic factors 54–5
Standards assessment 124
Supplier-induced demand 48
Surgical outcomes 55–6
Surgical specialties 43
Taxation 32, 57, 142, 203
  cost of 74–9
Technology advances 203–4
Technology assessment 47
Total quality management (TQM) 129
Two-class approach 72

Uninsured persons 213–18
  characteristics of 215–16
  estimates of 213
  health consequences 218
  reasons for lack of coverage 216–17

Upper gastrointestinal tract endoscopy 117
USA
  comparison with Canada 58, 85
  future directions 58–9
  health care rationing 48–50
  health care system 25
  health care system reform proposals 197–273
  medical manpower growth 42–4
  services *vs.* pensions 104–7
Utilisation research institutes 47

Vertical equity 2

Waiting lists 48, 50, 53

Index compiled by Geoffrey C. Jones